Dental Implantology Dictionary

Arun K. Garg, D.M.D.

GARG MULTIMEDIA GROUP, INC.

GARG MULTIMEDIA GROUP, INC.
1840 NE 153rd Street
North Miami Beach, FL 33162

www.ImplantSeminars.com

Second Edition

ISBN: 978-0-9820953-4-8

Interior design by Robert Mott & Associates
www.RobertMottDesigns.com

*"**Dentist:** (a person) who, while putting metal into your mouth, pulls coin out of your pocket."* — AMBROSE BIERCE

Americans, obsessed with good health and beauty, are now regularly coping with dental problems. With an estimated two out of three Americans having at least one missing tooth, implants have become the preferred tooth-replacement option.

Dental Implant Surgery is one of the safest, most precise and predictable procedures in dentistry, yet Dental Implant Surgery is still in its infancy.

The study of Dental Implantology involves a whole new nomenclature. It is so new, that many terms can be easily misunderstood, and when a term is misunderstood, entire concepts are misunderstood. Because of the precise nature of implantology, this can be disastrous.

This dictionary was produced by a longtime professional in the field. This ensures a high dgree of professional reliability. It won't be filled with terms that will impede your quick access to the understanding you really need.

However, this is such a dynamic and evolving field that although current at the time of printing, the *Dental Implantology Dictionary*—unlike other dictionaries in other fields—may have terms that have changed or been added even after we've gone to print.

In this case, please send me any terms you feel were left out for future incorporation. Likewise, please send any terms you feel have changed.

We hope you find the *Dental Implantology Dictionary* useful.

—Dr. Arun K. Garg

A

Aberrant: deviating from the norm or the usual.

Abrade: to grind, rub, scrape, or wear away the surface of a part by friction.

Abrasion: a surface or a part worn away by natural or artificial means.

Abscess: an enclosed collection of pus on the body as a result of the body's defensive reaction to an infection. Most abscesses can occur anywhere in the body.

Absorbable: *See*: BIOABSORBABLE.

Absorption: the reception of substances through, by, or into biological tissue.

Abutment: the portion of an implant or implant component(s) above the neck of the implant that serves to support and/or retain a fixed, fixed-detachable, or removable dental prosthesis.

Abutment attachment: a mechanical device for the fixation, retention, or stabilization of an implant-borne dental prosthesis.

Abutment clamp: 1. any device used for positioning a dental implant abutment upon a dental implant body. 2. forceps used to assist in the positioning of an abutment on the implant platform.

Abutment connection: a procedure for securing an abutment to an implant.

A

Abutment level impression: the impression of an abutment either directly (using conventional impression techniques) or indirectly (using an abutment impression coping). *See*: IMPLANT LEVEL IMPRESSION.

Abutment screw: a screw used to secure the abutment to the implant, usually torqued to a final seating position.

Abutment selection: the decision during prosthodontic treatment concerning the type of abutment used for the restoration, based on implant angulation, interarch space, soft tissue (mucosal) height, planned prosthesis, occlusal factors (e.g., opposing dentition, parafunction), and esthetic and phonetic considerations.

Abutment swapping: *See*: PLATFORM SWITCHING.

Abutment transfer device: *See*: ORIENTATION JIG.

Access hole: the channel in a screw-retained implant prosthesis which receives the abutment or prosthetic screw, usually through the occlusal or lingual surface of the prosthesis.

Accessory ostium: occasional opening of the maxillary sinus either into the infundibulum or directly in the wall of the middle meatus. *See*: OSTIUM (MAXILLARY SINUS).

Acellular: having no cells.

Acellular dermal allograft: a substitute for autogenous soft tissue grafts in root coverage procedure which replaces lost dermis and is used as a synthetic or biosynthetic material. Also referred to as skin grafts.

A

Acid-etched implant: external surface of an implant body modified by the chemical action of an acidic medium intended to enhance osseointegration.

Acid-etched surface: an implant surface treated with acid to increase the surface area by subtraction. *See:* SUBTRACTED SURFACE.

Acrylic resin: a self-cured or heat-cured plastic consisting of monomers (usually liquid) and polymers (usually powders).

Actinobacillus actinomycetemcomitans: a species of gram-negative, facultatively anaerobic, spherical or rod-shaped bacteria; frequently associated with some forms of human periodontal disease as well as subacute and chronic endocarditis; occurs with actinomycetes in actinomycotic lesions.

Actonel: an oral bisphosphonate; brand name for active ingredient risedronate sodium; used to treat Paget's disease of the bone, and to prevent and treat postmenopausal osteoporosis and glucocorticoid-induced osteoporosis in men and women. Several cases of Bisphosphonate-related osteomyelitis (BON, also referred to as osteonecrosis of the jaw) have been associated with the use of the oral bisphosphonates [Fosamax (alendronate), Actonel (risedronate) and Boniva (ibandronate)] for the treatment of osteoporosis; these patients may have had other conditions that could put them at risk for developing BON.

Added surface: *Syn*: Additive surface treatment; alteration of an implant surface by addition of material. *See*: SUBTRACTED SURFACE, TEXTURED SURFACE.

Additive surface treatment: *See*: ADDED SURFACE.

A

Adduct: to pull or draw medially.

Adhesion: the sticking together of dissimilar materials.

Adjustment: a modification of a restoration of a tooth or of a prosthetic after insertion in the mouth.

Adsorption: adhesion of molecules to solid or liquid surfaces.

Ailing implant: general term for an implant affected by implant mucositis, without bone loss; an implant with a history of bone loss. *See:* Peri-implant mucositis, Peri-implantitis.

Ala nasi: the wings of the nose.

Ala-tragus line: a line extending from the midpoint of the tragus to the nasal wings.

Algipore: a biological HA derived from calcifying maritime algae.

Alkaline phosphatase: a hydrolase enzyme used to remove phosphate groups from many types of molecules, including nucleotides, proteins, and alkaloids.

Allogenic: transplantation tissues of the same species but antigenically different.

Allogenic graft: tissue transplanted between members of the same species; a homograft. *See*: ALLOGRAFT.

Allograft: *Syn*: Allogenic graft; graft tissue from genetically dissimilar members of the same species. Three types exist: frozen, freeze-dried bone allograft (FDBA), and demineralized freeze- dried bone allograft (DFDBA). Allograft bone is processed and prepared from tissue banks. *See:* HOMOGRAFT, ALLOPLAST).

Alloplast: *Syn*: Alloplastic graft; synthetic, inorganic material used as a bone substitute or as an implant; a relatively inert synthetic material, generally metal, ceramic, or polymeric, used to construct, reconstruct, or augment tissue. *See*: IMPLANT.

Alloplastic graft: *See*: ALLOPLAST; graft of a relatively inert synthetic material.

Alloplastic material: relatively inert synthetic material, usually metal, ceramic, or polymeric.

Aluminum oxide: a metallic oxide. 1. Alpha Single Crystal: an inert, highly biocompatible, strong ceramic material from which some endosseous implants are fabricated. 2. Polycrystal: constituent of dental porcelain used to increase viscosity and strength.

Aluminum oxide (alpha single crystal): an inert, strong, highly biocompatible ceramic material from which endosseous implants are fabricated through crystal culture techniques.

Aluminum oxide (polycrystal): a fused A1203 biocompatible material.

Alveolar: pertaining to an alveolus. *See*: ALVEOLUS.

Alveolar augmentation: a surgical procedure designed to enlarge the morphology of a ridge. *See*: AUGMENTATION.

Alveolar bone: *See*: BONE; the portion of the jawbone that retained or retains teeth.

Alveolar crest: the most coronal portion of the alveolar process.

Alveolar defect: a deficiency in the contour of the alveolar ridge. The deficiency can be in the vertical (apicocoronal) and/or horizontal (buccolingual, mesiodistal) direction.

Alveolar distraction osteogenesis: *See*: DISTRACTION OSTEOGENESIS.

Alveolar mucosa: *Syn*: Lining mucosa; mucosa covering the alveolar process apical to the mucogingival junction, consisting of a nonkeratinized epithelium lining, a connective tissue that is loosely attached to the periosteum and movable; the mucous membrane covering the basal part of the alveolar process, continuing without demarcation into the vestibular fornix and the mouth's floor. *See*: ORAL MUCOSA.

Alveolar nerve: a terminal of the mandibular nerve that passes through the lower teeth, periosteum and gingiva of the mandible and finally to the skin of the chin and the mucous membrane of the lower lip. *See:* INFERIOR ALVEOLAR, INFERIOR DENTAL NERVE.

Alveolar process: the portion of the maxillae or mandible forming the dental arch and serving as a bony investment for the teeth; the compact and cancellous portion of bone surrounding and supporting the teeth. *See*: ALVEOLAR RIDGE, RESIDUAL RIDGE, RIDGE.

Alveolar recess: a cavity formed in the maxillary sinus floor formed by a septum. *See*: SEPTUM (MAXILLARY SINUS).

Alveolar reconstruction: surgical procedure designed to reshape or restore the alveolar ridge; alveoloplasty.

Alveolar ridge: the bony ridge of the maxillae or mandible containing the alveoli (teeth sockets); the remainder of the alveolar process after the teeth are removed. *See*: RESIDUAL RIDGE, RIDGE.

Alveolar ridge augmentation: *See*: AUGMENTATION.

Alveolar ridge resorption: *See*: RIDGE RESORPTION.

Alveolectomy: removal of a portion of the alveolar process, usually performed to achieve acceptable bone contour. *See*: OSTECTOMY.

Alveoloplasty: conservative contouring of the alveolar process to achieve acceptable ridge morphology. *See*: OSTEOPLASTY.

Alveolus: the socket in the bone in which a tooth is attached via the periodontal ligament; tooth socket.

Amorphous: free of crystalline structure.

Amoxicillin: an antibiotic effective against different bacteria found in and around the oral cavity including but not limited to such as Haemophilus influenzae, Neisseria gonorrhoea, Escherichia coli, Pneumococci, Streptococci, and certain strains of Staphylococci, particularly infections of the middle ear, tonsillitis, throat infections, laryngitis, bronchitis, and pneumonia. Amoxicillin is also used in treating urinary tract infections, and some skin infections.

Analgesic: a chemical that generally relieves pain without causing the patient to lose consciousness.

Analog (Analogue): *Syn*: Replica. a replica of an implant, abutment or attachment mechanism, usually incorporated within a cast for a prosthetic reconstruction; an implant replica on the laboratory bench used for purposes of prosthetic reconstruction.

Anatomy: branch of science that describes the morphology of organs; the art associated with separating the parts of an organism in order to determine the position, relations, structure, and function of those parts.

Anesthesia: absence of sensation to stimuli.

Angiogenesis: formation and differentiation of new blood vessels.

Angle, E. H.: occlusal conditions classified by anteroposterior relationships (Class 1, normal; Class 2, bilateral or partial protrusion of the maxilla; Class 3, protrusion of the mandible).

Angled abutment: a prosthetic coupling component of an implant (available in a variety of angles, up to 35 degrees), which is specially designed to be fitted with a crown or other anchorage attachment. *See*: ANGULATED ABUTMENT.

Angled implant: allows for implant placement within available bone while the restorative platform is located at optimal esthetic angle.

Angular cheilitis: inflammation of the corners of the mouth, frequently caused by bite over closure and sometimes by riboflavin deficiency.

Angulated abutment: *Syn*: Angled abutment; abutment with a body which is not parallel to the long axis of the implant. It is used when the implant is at a different inclination in relation to the proposed prosthesis; the portion of an endosteal implant that deviates from its long axis as it passes permucosally to serve as an anchorage device for a crown. *See*: NONANGULATED ABUTMENT.

Animal model: a laboratory animal used for medical research because it has specific characteristics, based on its breed and species, that can be affected similar to a human afflicted by a specific disease or disorder. Can be created by transferring genes into them.

Anisotropic surface: Surface with a directional pattern. *See*: ISOTROPIC SURFACE.

Ankylosis: bony consolidation in a joint between a tooth or implant and the jaw (see osseointegration); stiffness of a joint which is caused by disease or by surgery; the joining or union of distinct bones or separate hard parts to form one bone or part.

Anneal: to heat and then cool (metals or glass) by a slow process to prevent brittleness, to add toughness, and to maintain pliability.

Anodization: is an electrolytic passivation process used to increase the thickness of the natural oxide layer on the surface of metal to deter tarnish or corrosion. Anodization changes the microscopic texture of the surface and can change the crystal structure of the metal near the surface.

Anterior: the forward part or front part in anatomy.

Anterior loop: an extension of the inferior alveolar nerve, anterior to the mental foramen, and prior to exiting the mandibular canal.

Anterior nasal spine: *See*: NASAL SPINE.

Anteroposterior spread (AP spread): the distance from the center of the most anterior implant to a line joining the distal aspects of the most distal implants; a measurement which provides a guideline for the amount of acceptable cantilever within the bilateral distal extensions of an implant-supported prosthesis.

Antibiotic: substance produced by fungi that is able to inhibit bacterial growth used to treat infections caused by bacteria and other microorganisms.

Antirotation: a feature or characteristic that prevents the rotation of two joint components.

Antirotation component: a component of the implant body—hexagonal, tapered (Morse), or with some other internal design—placed to prevent unwanted abutment rotation.

Antral floor: bony floor of the maxillary sinus cavity, typically lower than the nasal floor and tending to be wider.

Antral mucosa: *See*: SCHNEIDERIAN MEMBRANE.

Antrum: based on Greek *antron*, meaning "cave"; a cavity or chamber within the bone. *See*: SINUS.

Antrum of Highmore: *See*: MAXILLARY SINUS.

Apatite: calcium phosphate; the mineral component of teeth and bones.

Aperture: an opening or hole.

Apex: the highest point or tip.

Apex region (or apical region): the area surrounding the root tips of teeth.

Aphagia: the inability to swallow.

Aphasia: the inability to speak.

Apical: referring to the apex.

Apical (retrograde) peri-implantitis: *See*: IMPLANT PERIAPICAL lesion.

AP spread: the acronym for Anteroposterior spread.

Appliance: a general reference to a prosthesis, splint, stent, template, guide, or denture.

Apposition: a description of the relationship of two parts when the parts are placed together or co-adapted.

Approximation: near or adjacent; the process of drawing parts together.

Arch form: the shape of the arch when viewed from above or below; the shape may be square, oval, round, or tapering, or some combination.

Arch length discrepancy: a reference to the differences between maxillary and mandibular arch forms, widths, lengths, and other dimensions.

Artery: a vessel that carries blood high in oxygen content away from the heart to the farthest reaches of the body.

Articulation: the natural relationship between upper and lower teeth in both static and dynamic function. Artificial articulation is the use of a mechanical device that simulates the movements of the temporomandibular joint, permitting the orientation of casts so as to duplicate or simulate various positions or movements of the patient.

Articulator: a complex or simple mechanical device used to simulate the jaws and their movements in order to fabricate a prosthesis.

Artifact: a foreign object revealed in the tissues through the use of diagnostic imaging or during palpation or during surgery.

Asepsis: prevention of contact with microorganisms; the state of the surgical field desirable for implant surgery.

Asleep: term used to describe a non-pathologic implant left submerged.

Asymmetry: a lack of balance or sameness.

Atrophic: characterized by atrophy, in other words, by a decrease in the size of the ridge because of resorption of the bone.

Atrophy: decrease in size of a cell, organ, tissue, or part. *See*: DISUSE ATROPHY, RIDGE ATROPHY.

Attached gingiva: part of the gingiva extending from the base of the sulcus to the mucogingival junction around teeth. The gingiva is "attached" to bone by the periosteum; to cementum by the gingival fibers; and to cementum, enamel, or dentin by the epithelial attachment. Alternately, the portion of the gingiva extending from the dental cervical margin to the alveolar mucosa; it is fairly dense, tightly bound to the underlying periosteum, tooth, and bone.

Attachment: a mechanical device for the fixation, retention, and stabilization of a dental prosthesis; the attachment may consist of one part or several parts; it is made of metal, plastic, or other materials.

Attachment device: *See*: ATTACHMENT.

Attachment screw: a threaded device used to fasten prostheses to implants, driven in or removed by using a specially designed driver, which is inserted in a geometric pattern in its widened head.

Attrition: the grinding or wearing down or away of hard issues as a result of functional friction.

Augmentation: placing autogenous or alloplastic materials in an attempt to correct deficiencies in the bone; alternately, the placement of a graft or any procedure that attempts to correct a soft tissue or hard tissue deficiency. *See*: BONE AUGMENTATION.

Auricular prosthesis: a device that artificially replaces all or part of an ear.

Autocrine: secretion of a chemical substance, such as hormones and growth factors, that stimulate the secretion within the cell itself.

Autogenous: self-generated.

Autogenous bone graft: bone harvested from one site and transplanted to another site in the same individual.

Autogenous graft: *Syn*: Autograft, Autologous graft; tissue taken from one site and transplanted to another site in the same individual.

Autograft: a graft taken from one part of the patient's body and transplanted to another part. *See*: AUTOGENOUS GRAFT.

Autologous: *See*: AUTOGENOUS.

Autologous graft: *See*: AUTOGENOUS GRAFT.

Available bone: a reference to that portion of an edentulous ridge which is available for the predictably stable insertion of an endosseous implant.

Avascular: lacking blood vessels.

Avascular necrosis: cell death which has occurred due to loss of blood supply.

Avulsion: a traumatic or surgical separation of a body part from its anatomic site.

Axial inclination: a reference to the alignment of the long axis of a tooth to a horizontal plane.

Axial loading: natural forces of function which are directed on the long axis of a tooth or implant; a reference, most often, to any force applied in the direction of the long axis of an implant. *See*: NONAXIAL LOADING.

Balanced occlusion: the simultaneous contact of the upper and lower teeth on the right and left and in the anterior and posterior areas in centric and eccentric positions within the functioning range; used primarily to ensure alignment of dentures or prosthetics.

Bar: *Syn*: Connecting bar; a type of connector between two or more implants or teeth, used to provide retention, stability, and/or support for a prosthesis.

Barium sulfate (BaSO4): finely ground radiopaque powder used in the construction of a radiographic template.

Bar overdenture (implant): a removable partial or complete denture, which may be either implant-supported or implant-tissue-supported. Implants in this type of reconstruction are connected with a bar incorporating attachment mechanisms for retention and support of the prosthesis.

Barrier membrane: *Syn*: Occlusive membrane; a device which helps to confine a grafted area, thus preventing movement or loss of grafting material and controls the growth of undesirable cells into a site with or without a graft material.

Basal bone: refers to the portion of the jawbone not including the alveolar processes. *See*: BONE.

Base metal: any metal that fails to resist a corrosive or oxidizing agent.

Basic multicellular unit (BMU): refers to a functional unit consisting of cellular elements responsible for bone formation and resorption (i.e., remodeling).

Basket endosteal dental implant: generally, a perforated or fenestrated cylindrical endosteal implant which has been designed to permit bone growth within its basket.

Beading: the placement of small balls or other devices for the adhesion of acrylic, cement, or other materials to a prosthesis.

Bending stress: refers to stress forces caused by a load that tends to bend an object. *See*: STRESS.

Bevel: a slanted edge.

BIC: *Acronym*: Bone-to-Implant Contact.

Bicortical stabilization: the substantive engagement of an implant with the crestal cortical bone of the edentulous ridge and the cortical bone of the base of the mandible or the floor of the maxillary sinus or floor of the nasal cavity. This term may also apply to the engagement of the facial and lingual cortices or any two cortices by an implant.

Bifid: split or double-headed.

Bifurcation: splitting into two parts (for example, a split at the point of mandibulomental separation).

Bilateral: referring to two sides.

Bilateral stabilization: *See*: CROSS-ARCH STABILIZATION.

Bimaxillary protrusion: a reference to the pronation of both jaws.

B

Bioabsorbable: *Syn*: Absorbable; the property of a material that degrades and dissolves in vivo. Breakdown products from such material are incorporated into normal physiologic and biochemical processes (for example, bioabsorbable membranes or sutures).

Bioacceptability: *See*: BIOCOMPATIBLE.

Bioactive: having the quality of interfacial metabolism after implantation; having an effect on, or eliciting a response from, living tissue. *See*: BIOINERT.

Bioactive fixation: fixation or stabilization which involves the direct physical or chemical attachment mechanisms between biological materials and an implant surface at the ultra-structural level.

Bioactive glass: absorbable alloplastic material composed of the metal oxides SiO2, Na2O, and P2O5. It has the ability to form a chemical bond with living tissues and thereby to help stabilize a filled defect site and maintain a rigid scaffold upon which cells can migrate and grow.

Biocompatible: ability of a material to function without a negative host response (immune response or inflammation) in a specific application. In general, biocompatibility can be measured on the basis of allergenicity, carcinogenicity, localized cytotoxicity, and systemic responses; also used to refer to a material that has qualities which permit it to remain in a biologic environment successfully.

Biodegradable: a reference to the property of a material which causes it to breaks down when placed in a biologic environment. *See*: BIOABSORBABLE.

Bioinert: the property of a material that elicits no host response. *See*: BIOACTIVE.

Biointegration: the process by which living tissue bonds to the surface of a biomaterial or implant, which is independent of any mechanical interlocking mechanism. The term is often used to describe the bond of living tissue to hydroxyapatite-coated implants. *See*: OSSEOINTEGRATION. Such bonding implies that contact is established without interposition of nonbony tissue between implant surface coating and host-remodeled bone; thus, a bond between the materials is formed biochemically, at the light microscopic level.

Biologic width: a reference to the combined width of the epithelial tissues and connective tissues above the bone level; alternately, the combined apicocoronal height of connective tissue and epithelial attachment. Such width exists around teeth as well as around dental implants once the implants are exposed to the oral cavity.

Biomaterial: non-viable material used to replace part of a living system or to function in contact with a living system; additionally, the term used to described a relatively inert, naturally occurring, or manmade material which can be used to implant in or interface with living tissues or biologic fluids without resulting in untoward reactions with those tissues or fluids; such material can be used to fabricate devices designed to replace body parts or functions.

Biomechanical test: a test which measures the physical properties of any biomechanical device, device-tissue interface (e.g., bone-implant), or the properties of tissues themselves.

Biomechanics: the science of applying mechanical laws to living structures; the field of science dealing with the mechanical properties of biologic structures as well as the interaction between mechanical devices and living tissues, organs, and organisms.

Bioengineering: the application of engineering methods and techniques to solve issues in medicine and biology, including structure and movement, or the design of prosthetics.

B

Biofilm: a layer of extracellular matrix containing quiescent, non-proliferating micro-organisms.

Biomimetic: able to replicate or imitate a body structure (anatomy) and/or function (physiology).

Biopsy: an evaluation and diagnosis of tissues removed from a living body.

Bioresorbable: *See*: RESORBABLE.

Bisphosphonate: an oral antiresorptive medicine which stops or slows the natural process that dissolves bone tissue, resulting in maintained bone density and strength. Note: Use of these medications has recently been linked to cases of jaw bone decay or osteonecrosis of the jaw (ONJ). ONJ or "dead jaw" is a rare bone disease in which the jaw bone deteriorates and dies. The discovery of this link was published in the Journal of Oral and Maxillofacial Surgeons.

Bite raising: a term used to refer to increasing the occlusal all-vertical dimension.

Black space: *See*: BLACK TRIANGLE.

Black triangle: *Syn*: Black space; a condition resulting from papilla missing or not totally filling the embrasure space.

Blade endosteal dental implant: *See*: BLADE IMPLANT.

Blade implant: an endosteal implant consisting of an abutment, cervix, and body (or infrastructure) that is buccolingually thin and has fenestrations to permit the ingrowth of bone/connective tissue for purposes of anchorage. Laminar endosseous implant designed to be placed within the bone in a surgically prepared thin groove.

Blanching: making white or pale, usually in reference to pen-implant or periodontal soft tissue (for example, during prosthetic try-in/insertion).

Bleeding on probing: bleeding that is induced by gentle manipulation of the tissue at the depth of the gingival sulcus, or interface between the gingiva and a tooth with a periodontal probe. The dentist records this in order to determine the periodontal health of a patient.

Block graft: graft consisting of a monocortical piece of autogenous bone (for example, chin or ramus) or a piece of bone replacement graft, usually stabilized in the recipient site with screws.

Block out: eliminating harmful undercuts from human bone or study casts using surgery or putty-like materials.

Blood cell: any of the cell types, red, white or platelet normally found in blood. In mammals are anucleate as they mature in order to provide more space for hemoglobin.

Blood clot: a semisolid mass in the bloodstream result from coagulation of the blood, primarily from platelets and fibrin.

BMP: *Acronym*: Bone morphogenetic protein.

BMU: *Acronym*: Basic multicellular unit.

Boil out: the elimination of wax using elevated temperatures.

Bond: a force that hold units of matter together.

Bone: the material of the skeleton of most vertebrate animals; the tissue constituting bones; the hard portion of the connective tissue constituting the majority of the skeleton. Bone consists of an inorganic component (67%, minerals such as calcium phosphate) and an organic component (33%, (collagenous matrix and cells). 1. Alveolar bone: bony portion of the mandible or maxilla in which the roots of the teeth are held by periodontal ligament fibers. Alveolar bone is formed during tooth development and eruption. 2. Basal bone: bone of the mandible or maxilla, excluding the alveolar bone. 3. Bundle bone: type of alveolar bone, so called because of the continuation into it of the principal (Sharpey's) fibers of the periodontal ligament. 4. Cancellous bone: *Syn*: Medullary bone, Spongy bone, Trabecular bone. Bone in which the trabeculae form a three-dimensional latticework with the interstices filled with bone marrow. 5. Cortical bone: *Syn*: compact bone. The noncancellous hard and dense portion of bone that consists largely of concentric lamellar osteons and interstitial lamellae. 6. Lamellar bone: the normal type of mature bone, organized in layers (lamellae) that may be concentrically arranged (compact bone) or parallel (cancellous bone). 7. Woven bone: *Syn*: Nonlamellar bone, Primary bone, Primitive bone, Reactive bone. Immature bone encountered where bone is healing or being regenerated.

Bone atrophy: bone resorption manifested externally by morphologic change and internally by changes in density; decrease in the dimensions of bone due to its resorption.

Bone augmentation: the application of one of a variety of surgical procedures to enhance the dimensions of a potential operative site; placement of an autogenous graft and/or a bone replacement graft, or any procedure that corrects a hard tissue deficiency.

Bone, basal: the part of the mandible and maxillae from which the alveolar process develops.

Bone biopsy: a portion of bone under pathological examination for diagnosis.

Bone, bundle: the bone that forms the immediate attachment of the numerous bundles of collagen fibers incorporated into bone.

Bone, cancellous: the bone that forms a trabecular network and surrounds marrow spaces that may contain either fatty or hematopoietic tissue; this bone lies subjacent to the cortical bone and makes up the main portion (bulk) of a bone; also referred to as spongiosa, spongy bone, supporting bone, medullary bone, trabecular bone.

Bone cell: bone-forming osteoblasts, mature osteocytes, and degenerative osteoclasts which resorb. *See:* BONE.

Bone, compact: hard, dense bone constituting the outer, cortical layer and consisting of an infinite variety of penosteal bone, endosteal bone, and Haversian system.

Bone condenser: *See*: OSTEOTOME.

Bone, curettage: gentle moving of medullary bone by use of hand instruments to create an implant receptor site or to remove diseased intraosseous tissue; surgical shaving or smoothing of the bone surface.

Bone density: 1. Clinical: Tactile assessment of bone quality reflecting the percentage of calcified bone to marrow, determined during osteotomy preparation. Usually classified from Dl (dense) to D4 (porous). Other classifications exist. 2. Histological: The "density" is calculated from the percentage of all bone tissue constituted by mineralized bone. 3.

Radiographic: An estimate of the total amount of bone tissue (as bone mineral) in the path of one or more x-ray beams, as measured by Hounsfield Units. When in quotes, "density" is as defined in absorptiometry. The term does not mean *density* as used in physics.

Bone derivative: one of the substances extracted from bone (for example, such as bone morphogenetic proteins).

Bone expander: *See*: OSTEOTOME.

Bone expansion: immediate or longer-term increases of bone width via surgery. *See*: RIDGE EXPANSION.

Bone factor: the relationship between osteogenesis and Osteolysis.

Bone graft: *Syn*: Osseous graft; autogenous bone used for grafting.

Bone grafting: a surgical procedure performed to establish additional bone volume, using autogenous bone and/or a bone replacement graft, prior to or simultaneously with implant placement. *See*: BONE GRAFT, BONE REPLACEMENT GRAFT, BONE SUBSTITUTE.

Bone growth factors: histochemicals, proteins, and enzymes that have been shown to be responsible for assisting or enhancing bone growth (for example, bone morphogenic protein [BMP]).

Bone implant interface: *See*: IMPLANT INTERFACE.

Bone loss (implant): Physiologic or pathologic bone resorption around an implant. *See*: CRESTAL BONE LOSS, EARLY CRESTAL BONE LOSS, IMPLANT PERIAPICAL LESION, PERI-IMPLANTITIS.

Bone marrow: Soft spongy tissue found in the center of bone that contains fat and/or hematopoietic tissues; the soft, highly vascularized tissue within the intermedullary space responsible for hematopoiesis and osteogenetic cells.

Bone mass: a term used to reference the amount of bone tissue, frequently estimated by absorptiometry, and viewed as volume minus the marrow cavity. Quotations around the definition are used to distinguish it from the term "mass" in physics.

Bone matrix: the intercellular element of bone; the matrix consists of osteo-collagenous fibers, which are embedded in an amorphous substance as well as inorganic salts.

Bone milling: process by which particulate harvested bone is progressively transformed into smaller particles.

Bone morphogenetic protein (BMP): osteogenic protein produced by osteoblasts and stored in bone, capable of causing growth in nonosseous tissues. *See*: OSTEOINDUCTION.

Bone morphogenetic protein 2 (BMP-2): a poly-peptide protein known to stimulate secretion of alpha 1, a core-binding factor. It is an important factor in the development of bone and cartilage.

Bone morphogenetic protein 7 (BMP-7): member of the family of super proteins TGF-β it plays a key role in the transformation of mesenchymal cells into bone and cartilage. It's inhibitors are noggin and a similar protein, chordin,

Bone necrosis: *See*: Osteonecrosis.

Bone quality: an assessment of bone based on its density.

Bone regeneration: the renewal and/or repair of bone tissue.

Bone remodeling: *See*: REMODELING (BONE).

Bone replacement graft: a hard tissue graft (though not autogenous bone) used to stimulate new bone formation in an area where bone formerly existed.

Bone resorption: Bone loss as a result of osteoclastic activity.

Bone sounding: *See*: RIDGE SOUNDING.

Bone spreader: *See*: OSTEOTOME.

Bone substitute: a bone graft consisting of alloplastic material.

Bone tap: *See*: TAP.

Bone-to-implant contact (BIC): direct contact between surfaces of bone and implant at the light microscope level. *See*: PERCENTAGE BONE-TO-IMPLANT CONTACT.

Bone trap: refers to a device employed to harvest bone chips, osseous coagulum.

Bone trephine: *See*: TREPHINE.

Bony ankylosis: osseous joining; concerning teeth, a reference to periodontal tissue loss, and cementum bonding to alveolus.

Brittle: fragile, non-elastic, and fracture-prone.

Buccal index: an recorded impression of the facial aspect of teeth, with reference to a cast.

Bundle bone: *See*: BONE.

Button implant: *See*: MUCOSAL INSERT, INTRAMUCOSAL INSERT.

C

CAD/CAM: *Acronym*: computer-aided design/computer-aided manufacturing. Computer-assisted design; manufacturing accomplished through computer-assistance; a milling accomplished through computer control or stereolithography.

Calcium carbonate (CaCO3): *See*: CORALLINE.

Calcium phosphate: 1. Types of minerals (usually from surrounding bone or blood supply) required for mineralization of new bone within a graft site 2. Class of ceramics (with varying calcium-to-phosphorous ratios) used as a grafting material due to their ability to directly bond with bone *See*: ALLOPLAST.

Calcium sulfate (CaSO4): *See*: Dental stone, Plaster; Plaster of Paris.

Caldwell-Luc: a surgical procedure which attempts to relieve chronic sinusitis by an incision into the canine fossa to improve the drainage of the maxillary sinus; also includes a nasal antrostomy. Named after American physician George Caldwell and French laryngologist Henry Luc.

Callus: tissue forming around fractured bone segments for maintaining structural integrity and facilitating the generation of bone.

Calvarial graft: bone harvested for a graft from the superior portion of the cranium. Most often, this graft is taken from the parietal region, usually the right side (non-dominant hemisphere) behind the coronal suture, approximately 3 cm lateral to the sagittal suture.

Calvarium: refers to the bones of the skull, specifically consisting of three layers, including outer (cortex), middle diploe (medullary), and inner (cortex).

Cancellous bone: *See*: BONE, CANCELLOUS.

Canine protected articulation: separation of the buccal segments during eccentric movements of the mandible caused by overlap of the canines.

Cantilever: a beam segment or bridge segment supported at only one end.

Cantilever fixed partial denture: a fixed bridge most often at the distal end with unsupported pontics.

Cartilage: mesenchyme-derived tissue from a protective medium which is both compliant and flexible.

Case report: diagnostic and treatment documentation describing patient progress and outcomes.

Case sequencing: for a patient undergoing dental implant therapy, this term refers to the order of treatment (for example, time of treatment related to healing and prosthodontic restoration).

Castable abutment: *Syn*: UCLA abutment; cast component fabricated by waxing a plastic burnout pattern with or without a prefabricated cylinder; used to fabricate a custom abutment for either a cement-retained or screw-retained prosthesis.

CAT: computerized axial tomography.

CAT scan: *Acronym*: Computed axial tomography scan.

CBCT Scanners: *See*: CONE BEAM COMPUTED TOMOGRAPHY.

Cellulitis: inflammation (purulent) of loose connective tissue.

Cement: a substance designed to bond (temporarily or permanently) prostheses to implants or natural teeth.

Cement-retained: refers to the use of cement for retention of a prosthesis to an abutment. *See*: SCREW-RETAINED.

Center of the ridge: the site of the linea alba.

Centric: pertaining to or situated at the center.

Centric occlusion: maximum intercuspation of teeth.

Centric relationship: when the condyles are in their most posterior positions in the glenoid fossa, this relationship is the most posterior one of the mandible to the maxillae.

Ceramic: afloplastic material used for bone grafting and to fabricate abutments and prostheses. *See*: ALLOPLAST.

Ceramics: strong, hard, brittle, and inert nonconductors of thermal and electrical energy; metal and oxygen compounds formed of chemically and biochemically stable substances; characterized by ionic bonding.

Cervix: *See*: IMPLANT NECK; the connection between the infrastructure of the implant with the abutment; the neck of the implant.

Chamfer: a beveled edge which connects two surfaces.

Chemotaxis: directed movement of a cell or organism along a chemical concentration gradient either toward or away from a chemical stimulus source. Also called chemotropism.

Chin graft: a mostly cortical bone graft which is harvested from the facial aspect of the symphyseal area of the mandible;

this area is located between the mental foramina, apical to the roots of the teeth; it is usually above the mandible's lower border.

Chisel: an instrument with a beveled cutting edge used for cutting or cleaving hard tissue.

Chlohexidine: $C_{22}H_{30}Cl_2N_{10}$, *Syn*: Chlorhexidine.

Chronic: a reference to a patient's condition which is long-standing and non-acute.

Chronic abscess: a long-standing collection of pus surrounded by fibrous tissue without signs of inflammation. Usually developing slowly.

Chronic infection: an infection that lasts for days, to months, to a lifetime and typically develop from acute infections.

Circumferential subperiosteal implant: *See*: SUBPERIOSTEAL IMPLANT.

Clamping force: when torque is used to screw two components together, elastic deformation of the screen can result: this result is known as clamping force. *See*: PRELOAD.

Clean technique: the use of sterile instruments, implants, grafts, and irrigation solution during a surgical procedure in a clinical setting., but while operating room level sterility is not achieved, the surgeons wear sterile gloves, and the surgeons and assistants wear non-sterile attire. Under such conditions, the patient may or may not be covered by sterile drapes. *See*: STERILE TECHNIQUE.

Clip: an overdenture element used for fixation to a bar; the element usually grasps by spring action and is composed of plastic or metal. *See*: BAR OVERDENTURE.

Closed tray impression: *Syn*: Indirect impression. This technique uses an impression coping with positioning features; a rigid elastic impression material is injected around these features. Once the impression is removed, the coping is unthreaded from the mouth and then connected to a laboratory analog; subsequently, it is repositioned into the impression before pouring. *See*: OPEN TRAY IMPRESSION.

Closure screw: *See*: COVER SCREW.

Coating: 1. Abutment: surface treatment for used to alter optical transmission characteristics. 2. Implant: a substance applied to all or a portion of the dental implant's surface.

Coatings: a technique for making implant substrates more biocompatible by covering them with layers of materials designed for this purpose.

Cohesion: molecular bonding; the joining or attraction of similar materials.

Cohort study: a longitudinal study conducted by choosing a cohort group exhibiting a specific characteristic and following this group over a specified time to discover related characteristics (presumably).

Col: an interdental gingival depression between the facial and lingual papillae and conforms to the shape of the interproximal area.

Collagen: the proteinaceous white fibers, often used in grafting procedures, which occupy over half of bone, muscle, and connective tissue. A molecule whose characteristics include a triple helical structure and a high content of certain substances, namely glycinc, proline and hydroxyproline. Collagen represents a major constituent of a number of anatomical elements, including connective tissue fibers, the organic matrix of bone, dentin, cementum, and basal laminas. Fibroblasts, chondroblasts, osteoblasts, and odontoblasts are used to synthesize collagen. The human body consists of several types of collagen, including Type I, which is one of the first products the body synthesizes during bone formation.

Collagen membrane: a bioabsorbable membrane composed of collagen (mainly Type I); membrane properties: semi-permeable, hemostatic and chemotactic, and tolerated well by surrounding tissues.

Collar: *See*: IMPLANT COLLAR.

Combination syndrome: a condition of significant maxillary anterior alveolar resorption when lower anterior teeth are present and the posteriors are absent.

Comfort cap: *See*: HYGIENE CAP.

Commercially pure titanium (CP- Ti): a metal alloy (99 wt.% titanium) commonly used for dental implants because of its biocompatibility. Oxygen amounts (from 0.18 to 0.40 wt.%) within the alloy determine its grade. Trace elements include less than 0.25 wt.% of iron, carbon, hydrogen, and nitrogen. *See*: TITANIUM, TITANIUM ALLOY.

Compact bone: dense bone of the outer layer or cortex. *See*: BONE.

Compatible: a reference to a high degree of interchangeability of prosthetic components between one implant system and another.

Complete arch subperiosteal implant: a subperiosteal implant which is designed for an arch that is completely edentulous.

Complete subperiosteal implant: *See*: SUBPERIOSTEAL IMPLANT.

Complication: a reversible or irreversible unfavorable condition.

Composite graft: a graft consisting of a combination of different materials.

Composite resin: a tooth-colored plastic mixture filled with a bisphenol A-glycidyl methacrylate BISMA or urethane dimethacrylate (UDMA), and an inorganic filler such as silicon dioxide silica. Primarily used to restore decayed areas, but also for cosmetic dental improvements of the color or shaping of the teeth.

Compression: refers to a force which is delivered to the surface of an object at right angles.

Compressive stress: an induced force that usually leads to the shortening or compression of a body or object when two forces are applied toward one another in the same straight line. *See*: STRESS.

Computed axial tomography (CAT scan): *See*: COMPUTED TOMOGRAPHY.

Computed tomography (CT): the use of x-rays to produce a digital description of an image for display on a computer monitor or on a film for diagnostic studies of internal body structures; the x-rays produce a series of scans along a single axis of a bodily structure to construct a three-dimensional, panoramic, or cross-sectional image of that structure.

Computer-aided design / computer-aided manufacturing (CAD/CAM): the use of computer-acquired or computer-generated data to prepare a physical object.

Computer-aided navigation: the use of high-resolution computed tomography for surgical placement of implants.

Cone Beam Computed Tomography (CBCT): a scanner which uses a cone shaped x-ray beam instead of a conventional linear fan beam to produce images of the bony structures of the skull; such scanners have been available for craniofacial imaging in Europe (since 1999) and the United States (since 2001).

Configuration: refers to the specific size and shape of an implant or an implant component.

Congenital: a condition which exists at or which dates from the birth an individual, of nongenetic etiology.

Connecting bar: a fixed bar connecting two or more permucosal extensions (for example, an integral part of the substructure of the ramus frame or subperiosteal implant). *See*: BAR.

Connective tissue: binding and supportive tissue composed of fibroblasts, primitive mesenchymal cells, collagen fibers, and elastic fibers; connective tissue is also composed of associated blood and lymphatic vessels, nerve fibers, and so on. Connective tissue is considered primary tissue, but it has many forms and functions, including support, storage, and protection. Its larger proportion of extracellular matrix makes it distinct from other types of tissue.

Connective tissue attachment: the mechanism by which connective tissue attaches to the tooth or the implant. Connective tissue fibers run parallel to the implant surface and compose the apical part of biologic width.

Connective tissue graft: also known as a subepithelial connective tissue graft, is a thin piece of tissue grafted from the roof of the mouth, or harvested from an adjacent areas, to augment attached gingiva around the tooth. The gingival graft is placed to cover an exposed portion of the root, to create a stable band of attached tissue around the root.

Consolidation period: *See*: DISTRACTION OSTEOGENESIS.

Contact osteogenesis: this term refers to the direct migration of bone-building cells; the migration takes place through the clot matrix to form new bone first on the implant surface. *See*: DISTANCE OSTEOGENESIS.

Contour: an object's outline, shape, or silhouette.

Contralateral: refers to the side opposite another side.

Contraindication: when a treatment would involve a greater-than-normal risk to the patient, based on a certain condition or factor, and is therefore not recommended. When the patient is at higher risk of complications and there is no circumstance important enough to undertake the risky treatment, the contraindication is called "absolute." If the patient is at higher risk of complications but these risks may be outweighed by other considerations or mitigated by other measures, the contraindications are called *relative.*

Coolant: an irrigating fluid used to reduce the heat generated during drilling in the alveolar bone.

Coping: a prefabricated (or custom) component which fits on an implant or on an abutment; a thimble made of metal, ceramic, or plastic to fit an abutment.

Coping screw: *See*: PROSTHETIC SCREW.

Coralline: ceramic used as a grafting material and made from the calcium carbonate skeleton of coral.

Coral-derived hydroxyapatite: a non-biodegradable structure derived from natural coral through a hydrothermic process used to promote bone ingrowth (osseointegration) into prosthetic implants. The high temperature used to create it also burn off proteins, preventing graft-versus-host disease (GVHD).

Corrode: a term used to refer to the chemical deterioration metal placed in a biologic or saline environment.

Cortical bone: the peripheral layer of compact osseous tissue; the average thickness of which is 2 mm. *See*: BONE, COMPACT).

Corticocancellous bone: a piece of bone that contains both cortical bone full of morphogenetic proteins, and cancellous bone, that functions as graft.

Corticotomy: a surgical procedure during which only the bony cortex is cut.

Countersink: enlarge an osteotomy in the coronal part using a specific drill to accommodate the implant platform.

Countersink drill: drill for enlarging the coronal part of an osteotomy.

Cover screw: *Syn*: Closure screw, Healing screw; a cap-type screw for sealing the platform of an implant during osseointegration.

Cover screw mill: device to remove excess bone growth over a cover screw.

CP-Ti: *Acronym*: Commercially pure titanium.

Crestal: pertaining to the most coronal portion of the ridge.

Crestal bone loss: resorption of the most coronal aspect of the ridge surrounding the implant neck.

Crestal implant placement: placing an implant with the edge of the platform at the crest of bone. 1. Subcrestal: placement with the edge of the platform apical to the crest of bone. 2. Supracrestal: placement with the edge of the platform coronal to the crest of bone.

Crestal incision: incision made at the crest of the edentulous ridge. *See*: MIDCRESTAL INCISION, MUCOBUCCAL FOLD INCISION.

Crest of the ridge: *See*: ALVEOLAR CREST.

Crevicular: a reference to the gingival crevice.

Crevicular epithelium: the nonkeratinized epithelium of the gingival crevice. *See*: SULCULAR EPITHELIUM.

Critical-sized defect: osseous defects of a size that will not heal during the lifetime of the organism may be termed critical size defects (CSDs).

Cross-arch stabilization: *Syn*: Bilateral stabilization; a form of stabilization resulting from resistance to dislodging or rotational forces when a prosthetic design uses implants and/or natural teeth on opposite sides of the dental arch and splinted together.

Crossbite: a form of malocclusion resulting from the mandibular teeth being buccal to the maxillary teeth.

Crossbite occlusion: an occlusion in which the mandibular teeth overlap the maxillary teeth.

Cross-sectional study: A type of study that involves the observation of a defined population at a single point in time or time interval.

Crown: the tooth portion protruding into the mouth for chewing; also a reference to a prosthetic replacement for such a structure.

Crown-implant ratio: ratio of crown height to the length of the implant when surrounded by bone; "crown height" is the extension from the most coronal bone-to-implant contact to the most coronal aspect of the prosthetic reconstruction which is connected to that implant.

Crown-root ratio: the mathematical ratio of crown length to root length.

CT: computerized tomography; connective tissue.

Cumulative success rate: percentage of implant success over time. *See*: SUCCESS RATE.

Cumulative survival rate: the percentage of implant survival over time. *See*: SURVIVAL RATE.

Curettage: Scraping or scooping infected or inflamed tissue, or cavity in teeth.

Curve of Spee: an anatomic curvature of the occlusal alignment of teeth, beginning at the tip of the lower canine, following the buccal cusps of the natural premolars and molars, and continuing to the anterior border of the ramus.

Custom abutment: a component machined or cast for a unique circumstance.

Cylinder (Cylindrical) implant: endosseous root-form, press-fit implant with parallel-sided walls; a threaded or press-fit round endosteal implant.

Cylinder root form: *See*: CYLINDER IMPLANT.

Cylinder wrench: device used to place an implant into its osteotomy and to tighten the implant after placement.

Cytokine: a category of signal line proteins and glycoproteins that, like hormones and neurotransmitters, are used extensively in cellular communication.

D

DBM: *Acronym*: demineralized bone matrix.

Debridement: exposing healthy tissue by removing foreign material and contaminated or devitalized tissue from or adjacent to a traumatic or infected lesion.

Decortication: removal, in whole or in part, of the bony cortex to induce bleeding and release of bone-forming cells from the marrow.

Definitive prosthesis: a dental prosthesis to be used over a prescribed period of time, or longterm.

Deglutition: swallowing.

Dehiscence: 1. Incomplete coverage or cleft-like absence of bone at localized areas of teeth or implants, extending for a variable distance from the crest. *See*: FENESTRATION. 2. Premature opening of primary soft tissue closures.

Dehiscence, implant: a break in the covering epithelium, resulting in an isolated area of an implant or bone exposed to the oral cavity.

Dehiscence, mandibular: extreme resorption of the mandible resulting in exposure of the inferior alveolar nerve so that bone no longer covers the roof of the mandibular, leaving soft tissue alone to separate the contents of the canal from the oral cavity.

D

Delayed loading: time of applying force on an implant after initial placement when prosthesis is attached or secured after a conventional healing period. *See*: EARLY LOADING.

Demineralization: mineral loss.

Demineralized bone matrix (DBM): a chemical process of mineral extraction resulting in a composite of collagenous proteins, noncollagenous proteins, and bone growth factors remaining.

Demineralized freeze-dried bone allograft (DFDBA): Collagen (mainly Type I) which remains after demineralization of freeze-dried bone allograft (FDBA).

Dense cortical bone: *See*: CORTICAL BONE.

Dental implant: a permucosal, biocompatible, and biofunctional device placed on or within the bone of the oral cavity to support fixed or removable prostheses; Iso definition: "A device designed to be placed surgically within or on the mandibular or maxillary bone to provide resistance to displacement of a dental prosthesis." (ISO 1942-5).

Dental implant body: portion of an endosteal blade or root form implant which is attached by the cervix to the abutment and designed to achieve intraosseous retention.

Dental plaster: *See*: DENTAL STONE.

Dental stone: alpha-form of calcium sulfate hemihydrate, not used as a grafting material. *See*: PLASTER.

Denture: artificial substitute for missing natural teeth and adjacent tissues, not necessarily a removable prosthesis, or a device to completely cover an arch. *See*: FIXED PROSTHESIS, REMOVABLE PROSTHESIS.

Denture adhesive: substance used to adhere a prosthesis to the mucosa.

Denture flange: that portion of the denture base which extends from the teeth to the vestibules; the denture margins.

Denture flask: metal container for fabricating acrylic prostheses.

De-osseointegration: loss of achieved osseointegration from peri-implantitis and/or occlusal overload.

Depassivation: loss or removal of a metal's surface oxide layer caused by local conditions that produce an acidic environment. *See*: Passivation.

Depth gauge: graduated instrument whose markings measure the vertical extent of an osteotomy.

Dermal graft: de-epithelialization and de-cellularized immunologically inert avascular connective tissue obtained from a cadaver.

Design (implant): form, shape, configuration, surface macrostructure, and micro-irregularities of the three-dimensional structure of an implant or component.

Device orientation: distraction device position, usually relative to the anatomical axis of bone segments for distracting.

DFDBA: *Acronym*: Demineralized freeze-dried bone allograft.

Diagnostic wax-up: lab procedure creating teeth in wax according to the planned restoration; used to evaluate the feasibility of a plan and to fabricate a radiographic template, a surgical guide, or laboratory guides.

Diarthrodial joint: an articulation that is freely moving.

Direct bone impression: a negative recording of jawbone that is surgically exposed, made usually used to fabricate a subperiosteal implant.

Direct impression: *See*: OPEN TRAY IMPRESSION.

Direction indicator: a device which is inserted into an osteotomy to assess its orientation or position relative to adjacent teeth and anatomic structures. This term is also used to verify and assist in achieving parallelism when the clinician is preparing multiple osteotomies.

Disc implant: an implant whose endosteal design consists of a thin, plate-like component which is placed into a horizontal osteotomy and attached to a post-like vertical component which protrudes permucosally.

Disclusion (disocclusion)**:** a reference to the separation of the teeth in opposing jaws.

Disk implant: a reference to a kind of endosseous implant which consists of a plate, a neck, and an abutment which is inserted into the edentulous ridge laterally.

Distance osteogenesis: a gradual process of bone healing which occurs from the edge of the osteotomy and towards the implant. In this process, bone does not grow directly on the implant surface. *See*: CONTACT OSTEOGENESIS.

Distraction: *See*: DISTRACTION OSTEOGENESIS

Distraction axis: the direction that the distal bone segment is distracted.

Distraction device: an appliance allowing gradual movement of bone segments away from each other incrementally.

Distraction osteogenesis: *Syn*: Osteodistraction; an invasive surgical technique which employs specialized instruments allowing bones to become lengthened as much as 500 mu per day. Formation of new soft tissue and bone between vascular bone surfaces which is created by an osteotomy and separated by gradual, controlled distraction. The process begins with the development of a reparative callus. Placing the callus under tension by stretching generates new bone. Distraction osteogenesis takes place in three sequential periods: 1. Latency: from bone division (i.e. surgical separation of bone into two segments) to the onset of traction, representing the time allowed for callus formation. 2. Distraction: from the application of gradual traction to the formation of bone segments and new tissue (regenerate tissue). 3. Consolidation: *Syn*: Fixation period; corticalization of the distraction regenerate, after the discontinuation of traction forces and segment movement.

Distraction parameters: the biological and biomechanical variables affecting the quality and quantity of bone formed during distraction osteogenesis.

Distraction period: *See*: DISTRACTION OSTEOGENESIS.

Distraction protocol: the sequence and duration of events during the process of distraction osteogenesis.

Distraction rate: daily total of distraction achieved.

Distraction regenerate: *See*: REGENERATE.

Distraction rhythm: the division rate of distraction osteogenesis based on the number of increments per day.

Distraction vector: a reference to the final direction and magnitude of traction forces which occur during distraction osteogenesis.

Distraction zone: *See*: REGENERATE.

Distractor: *See*: DISTRACTION DEVICE.

Disuse atrophy: inactivity resulting in diminution in dimension and/or density.

DO: *Acronym*: Distraction osteogenesis.

Dolder bar: a device used as a connector for multiple prosthetic elements, lending strength and retaining an overdenture or superstructure; often accompanied by special clips for grasping.

Donor site: an anatomic location used for contributions of tissues for a graft, including skin, mucosa, connective tissue, and bone.

Doxycycline: Doxycycline is a semi-synthetic tetracycline antibiotic developed in the early 1960s by Pfizer Inc. It works by slowing the growth of bacteria in the body. It is linked to both inhibiting tooth growth and tooth discoloration.

Drill extender: *See*: EXTENDER.

Drilling sequence: using specific drills in a specific step-by-step manner to prepare and increase the diameter of an osteotomy gradually prior to implant placement.

Ductility: the characteristic of a material ability to be strained plastically but suffering no permanent deformation from tension.

Dysfunction: an organ's or body part's inability to perform satisfactorily.

Dysthesia: a spontaneous or evoked condition in which the sense of touch is distorted and interpreted by the body as an unpleasant sensation. Sometimes perceived as painful such as burning, itching or prickling.

Early crestal bone loss: an event involving crestal bone loss around an implant during the first year after exposure to the oral environment; the loss is usually attributed at least in part to the formation of the biologic width.

Early implant failure: *Syn*: Primary implant failure; a root-form implant's failure due to the inability to establish osseointegration, resulting in mobility. *See*: LATE IMPLANT FAILURE.

Early implant placement: a treatment option in post-extraction sites of teeth in the anterior maxilla that involves the placement of an implant into a prepared socket immediately or soon after tooth extraction. Recent clinical studies show that dental implants placed directly into prepared sockets immediately after tooth extraction achieved successful results compared with late implantation.

Early loading: a reference to when force is applied to an implant soon after initial placement; a prosthesis is attached to the implant(s), earlier than after the conventional healing period. Loading time should be stated in days/weeks. *See*: DELAYED LOADING.

ECM: *Acronym*: Extracellular matrix.

Eccentric: a reference to a deviation from a central path.

Ectopic: generally, a reference to an object being out of place.

Edema: swelling which is secondary to the retention of fluid (e.g., lymph).

Edentulism: the absence or complete loss of all natural dentition.

Edentulous: refers to a patient who is experiencing a complete loss of all natural dentition.

Edentulous space: the space caused by a missing tooth that is located between teeth.

Elasticity: the characteristic allowing a structure or material to return to its original form after an external force is removed.

Elastic modulus: refers to the level of stiffness of a material within an elasticity range.

Elastomer: a material consisting of a base and catalyst that, after being mixed, sets into a supple but firm substance.

Electric discharge method (EDM): *Syn*: Spark erosion; a process involving the removal of precision metal via a series of electrical sparks which erode material from a work piece in a liquid medium under carefully controlled conditions.

Electron microscopy: the projection of images via electron beams thousands of times shorter than visible light, creating much greater magnification.

Elements: the fundamental aspects of an object or subject.

Elevator: multipurpose dental surgical tool used to elevate, prop up, strip, or scrape soft tissue and bones.

Elevator muscle: one of a group of muscles whose contraction closes the mandible.

Embrasure: a space between teeth (lesser = above the contact point; greater = below the contact point) that resembles a triangle in shape.

E

EMD: *Acronym*: Enamel matrix derivative.

Emergence angle: refers to the angle created by an imaginary extension of the long axis of an implant versus the corrected axis of the abutment.

Emergence profile: a reference to the contour of tooth (restored) or implant relative to surrounding tissues.

Emergence profile: a reference to the part of the axial contour of a tooth or prosthetic crown extending from the sulcus base beyond the margin of free soft tissue. This profile extends to the contour's height and produces a straight or convex profile in the apical third of the axial surface.

Enamel matrix derivative (EMD): a derivative of sterile protein aggregate from the enamel matrix, amelogenin, the precursor of developing teeth's enamel; these proteins are specially harvested from developing pig embryo teeth.

Endochondral ossification: is one of the two processes in which long bone tissue is formed, lengthened and healed. It requires a pre-existing cartilage model.

Endocrine: a function by which the body's chemical compounds, such as hormones, are secreted and get transported throughout the body to exact cell recipients through the bloodstream.

Endodontic endosteal implant: a (smooth or threaded) pin implant extending through the root into periapical bone and stabilizing a mobile tooth.

Endodontic implant: *Syn*: Endodontic pin, Endodontic stabilizer; a pin placed into a root canal, extending beyond the apex into the bone.

Endodontic pin: *See*: ENDODONTIC ENDOSTEAL IMPLANT, ENDODONTIC IMPLANT.

Endodontic stabilizer: *See*: ENDODONTIC IMPLANT.

Endodontic stabilizer implant: *See*: ENDODONTIC ENDOSTEAL IMPLANT.

Endosseous blade implant: *See*: BLADE IMPLANT.

Endosseous distractor: *Syn*: Intraosseous distractor; distraction device placed into the edentulous ridge and/or basal bone (maxilla or mandible) and used in distraction osteogenesis.

Endosseous implant: *Syn*: Endosteal implant; a device placed into the alveolar and/or basal bone of the maxilla or mandible to support a prosthesis.

Endosseous ramus implant: a type of implant that is used if the lower jawbone is too thin for a rootform or subperiosteal implant. A ramus implant is embedded in the jawbone in the back corners of the mouth (near the mandibular third molars) and near the chin. A thin metal bar around the top of the gum will then be fitted for prosthesis. Ramus implants can stabilize weak jaws and help prevent them from fracturing.

Endosteal dental implant abutment: *See*: ABUTMENT.

Endosteal dental implant body: *See*: DENTAL IMPLANT BODY.

Endosteal implant: a device placed within alveolar or basal bone to serve as a prosthetic abutment. *See*: ENDOSSEOUS IMPLANT.

Endosteal root form implant: that portion of an endosteal implant (blade or root form) attached by the cervix to the abutment and designed to achieve intraosseous retention.

Endosteum: tissue lining the medullary cavity of bone, composed of a single layer of osteoprogenitor cells and a small amount of connective tissue.

Endothelial progenitor cell: bone marrow-derived cells that circulate in the blood, have the ability to adhere or bind and contain LDL and differentiate into endothelial cells (the cells that make up the lining of blood vessels). There is evidence that circulating endothelial progenitor cells play a role in the repair of damaged blood vessels after a myocardial infarction. In fact, higher levels of circulating endothelial progenitor cells detected in the bloodstream predict for better outcomes and fewer repeat heart attacks.

Endotoxin: potentially toxic, natural compound found inside part of the outer membrane of the cell wall of Gram-negative bacteria.

Envelope flap: a flap elevated from a horizontal linear incision, parallel to the free gingival margin, with no vertical incision, either sulcular or submarginal.

Epidermal growth factor: a small, mitogenic protein that is involved in the regulation of normal cell growth, oncogenesis, and wound healing. It plays an important role in proliferation, and differentiation.

Epithelial attachment: the attachment mechanism of the junctional epithelium to the tooth or implant (i.e., hemidesmosomes). *See:* JUNCTIONAL EPITHELIUM; the continuation of the sulcular epithelium, joined to the tooth or adherent to implant structure, located at the base of the sulcus or pocket.

Epithelial cuff, implant: the band of tissue constricted around an implant cervix.

Epithelial implant: *See:* MUCOSAL INSERT.

Epithelialization: a reference to the kind of healing that takes place when epithelium grows over connective tissue.

Epithelium: the outer layer which covers the underlying connective tissue stroma; the tissue lining the intraoral surfaces and extending into the sulcus while adhering to the implant/tooth.

Epithelization: a reference to the secondary healing of epithelium.

Eposteal implant: a device which receives primary bone support by resting upon bone. *See:* SUBPERIOSTEAL IMPLANT.

ePTFE: *Acronym:* Expanded polytetrafluoroethylene.

Epulis: an oral pathologic condition that appears in the mouth as a tumor in the gingiva, is a mucosal hyperplasia that results from chronic low-grade trauma induced by a lesion caused by denture.

Erosion: the loss of hard or soft tissue resulting in a saucer-shaped configuration and caused by pathologic tooth wear; alternatively caused by trauma to the integument (an ulcer).

Erythrocyte: A mature red blood cell that contains hemoglobin and can carry oxygen to the body.

Esthetic: pertaining to beauty.

Esthetic zone: any dento-alveolar region which is visible during a patient's full smile. The relationship between gingiva, lips, and teeth determines a particular smile's description as high or low.

Etching: the use of acids or other agents (etchants) for increasing the surface area of an implant or other materials.

E

Etiology: contribution to the cause of a disease or condition.

Exclusion criteria: the characteristics preventing a participant entering a clinical trial. *See*: INCLUSION CRITERIA.

Exfoliation: loss of implanted materials or of implant-associated devices.

Expanded polytetrafluoroethylene (ePTFE): a polymer of tetrafluoroethylene which is stretched to allow fluid but not cells to pass; the polymer is used as a nonresorbable membrane in guided bone regeneration (GBR) and guided tissue regeneration (GTR).titanium reinforcement may or may not be used in conjunction with this polymer to maintain its shape. This polymer can also be used as a non-absorbable suture material.

Expanded polytetrafluoroethylene (ePTFE) membrane: surgical membrane for grafting believed to be an inert material for vascular prosthesis, made up of tetrafluoroethylene, and can be varied in porosity to fill clinical and biological requirements of its applications. Typically used to guide bone regenerative substances.

Expert witness: a person who has the training, education or experience on a particular subject and who is formally found to be qualified as an expert by a judge.

Exposure: 1. Implant: the dehiscence of soft tissue which leads to the exposure of the implant cover screw, neck, body, or threads. This is a colloquial term for stage-two surgery. 2. Barrier Membrane: the dehiscence of soft tissue which leads to the exposure of an occlusive membrane during the healing period.

Extender: a surgical component used as an intermediary between the handpiece or wrench and another component (e.g., drill, implant mount) in order to increase the reach of the latter part; a device for lengthening a bur, drill, or instrument.

External connection: a prosthetic interface external to the implant platform (e.g., an external hexagon) *See*: INTERNAL CONNECTION.

External hexagon: a connection interface of the platform of an implant which extends coronally and prevents rotation of attached components. *See*: INTERNAL HEXAGON.

External irrigation: method used during the drilling of osteotomies for the implants whereby a cooling solution is directed at the drilling bur, delivering the cooling solution at the entrance of the osteotomy; this cooling solution may be delivered through tubing connected to the handpiece and drilling unit; alternatively, it may be from a handheld system. *See*: INTERNAL IRRIGATION.

External oblique ridge: a smooth area on the buccal surface of the body of the mandible extending with diminishing prominence from the anterior border of the ramus both downward and forward to the region of the mental foramen;

the ridge changes only a small degree in size and direction over time, and is an important landmark in the design of a subperiosteal implant.

Extirpate: to remove an organ, body part, or neoplasm.

Extracellular matrix (ECM): a reference to any material produced by cells and excreted into the tissue's extracellular space. The matrix takes the form of both ground substance and fibrous elements, proteins involved in cell adhesion, and glycosaminoglycans, as well as other space-filling molecules. The matrix can serve as a scaffolding to hold tissues together; additionally, its form and composition help determine tissue characteristics.

Extraction socket: the alveolus resulting from tooth removal.

Extraction socket graft: *See*: RIDGE PRESERVATION.

Extraoral (external) distraction device: a device located outside the oral cavity and used in distraction osteogenesis; the bone segments are usually attached to percutaneous pins connected externally to device fixation clamps.

Extraosseous distractor: a device placed outside the edentulous ridge or basal bone of the maxilla or mandible and used in distraction osteogenesis.

Exudate: a reference to the fluids, cells, and cellular debris which have escaped from blood vessels and deposited in tissues or on tissue surfaces (frequently as a result of inflammation); fluid with a high content of protein which has escaped from blood vessels and deposited in tissues as a result of infection; pus; purulence.

Fabrication: structure or prosthesis construction.

Facebow: a device used to record the relationship of the maxillae to the opening axis of the mandible and to orient the casts in this same relationship to the opening axis of an articulator.

Facial augmentation implant prosthesis: a polymeric device which is shaped to restore a depressed or inadequate portion of the facial skeleton; it is implanted subperiosteally.

Facial moulage: impression of facial structures from elastomeric materials.

Failed implant: a mobile implant (failed to achieve or has lost osseointegration), or symptomatic in spite of osseointegration.

Failing implant: a general term for an implant that is progressively mobile; the implant may exhibit increased probing depth, purulence, but remains clinically stable. *See*: PERI-IMPLANTITIS.

Failure rate: percentage of failure in a study or clinical trial of a procedure or device (e.g., implant) not meeting the success criteria, or falling into the failure criteria, defined in the study protocol.

Fatigue: progressive weakening of a structure steady embrittlement and crack formation/propagation; breaking or fracturing of a material caused by repeated cyclic or applied loads below the yield limit.

Fatigue failure: fracture of a material from loading, resulting from stresses beyond tolerance; a structural failure caused by multiple loading when all loads lie below the structure's ultimate strength. Typically, such failures occur only after thousands or millions of loading episodes.

Fatigue fracture: structural failure caused by repetitive stresses, resulting in a slowly propagating crack to cross the material.

FDBA: *Acronym*: Freeze-dried bone allograft.

FEA: *Acronym*: Finite element analysis.

Fenestration: a single, isolated area where the root or implant surface is denuded of bone but not involving the crestal bone. *See*: DEHISCENCE.

Fibrinolysis: the process wherein a fibrin clot, the product of coagulation, is broken down. Its main enzyme plasmin cuts the fibrin mesh at various places, producing circulating fragments cleared by other proteases or by the kidney and liver.

Fibroblast: the cell type found within the connective tissue responsible for synthesis of collagen fibers and the ground substance of connective tissue.

Fibroblast growth factor (FGF): from the family of cytokines, FGFs promote the growth of new blood vessels from the pre-existing vasculature and give rise to granulation tissue, which fills up a wound space/cavity in the early wound-healing process. FGFs also have important roles in angiogenesis, neurogenesis and tumor growth. Humans have about 23 FGFs, with FGF-2 being the one use for regenerative treatments.

Fibro-integration: *See*: FIBRO-OSSEOUS INTEGRATION.

Fibronectin: a high-molecular-weight extracellular matrix glycoprotein that binds to receptor proteins, acting as binding sites for cell surface receptors. Fibronectin helps create a cross-linked network within the ECM by having binding sites for other ECM components. Fibronectin also serves as a plasma opsonin.

Fibro-osseous integration: incorporation of a blade implant into an osseous host site which is lined with fibrous tissue.

Fibro-osteal integration: *See*: FIBRO-OSSEOUS INTEGRATION.

Fibrosis: a reference to the process leading to formation of fibrous tissue (often degenerative).

Fibrous: composed of or containing fibers.

Fibrous encapsulation: layer of connective tissue in between implant and surrounding bone.

Fibrous integration: refers to soft tissue-to-implant contact; often refers to the interposition of healthy, dense, collagenous ligament tissue existing between a blade implant and bone transmitting load from the implant to the bone. *See*: FIBROUS ENCAPSULATION.

Finite element analysis (FEA): software technique used for the study of stresses and strains on mechanical parts. CAD software automatically generates the simulated mechanical loads for FEA measurements.

First-stage dental implant surgery: surgery during which the body of a two-piece implant is inserted.

Fissure: a cleft or groove.

Fistula: refers to the abnormal passage or communication (an abnormal epithelial-lined tract) between two internal organs or the passage leading from an internal organ to body surface. 1. Oroantral: an opening between oral cavity and maxillary sinus. 2. Orofacial: opening between the cutaneous surface of the face and oral cavity. 3. Oronasal: opening between the nasal cavity and oral cavity.

Fixation period: *See*: DISTRACTION OSTEOGENESIS.

Fixation screw: screw used to stabilize a block graft or a barrier membrane.

Fixation tack: *See*: TACK.

Fixed: nonremovable.

Fixed bridge: a prosthetic dental appliance replacing lost teeth and supported and held in position by attachments to natural teeth or implants nonremovably.

Fixed-detachable: prosthesis fixed to an implant or implants, but removable by the dentist. *See*: FIXED PROSTHESIS, CEMENT-RETAINED, HYBRID PROSTHESIS, IMPLANT-SUPPORTED PROSTHESIS, REMOVABLE PROSTHESIS, SCREW-RETAINED.

Fixed partial denture: *See:* FIXED BRIDGE.

Fixed prosthesis: restoration not removable by the patient; may be partial arch (FPD: Fixed partial denture), or complete arch (FCD: Fixed complete denture). *See*: DENTURE, REMOVABLE PROSTHESIS.

Fixed-removable: prosthesis fixed to an implant or implants, but removable by the dentist. *See*: FIXED PROSTHESIS, CEMENT-RETAINED, HYBRID PROSTHESIS, IMPLANT-SUPPORTED PROSTHESIS, REMOVABLE PROSTHESIS, SCREW-RETAINED.

F

Fixed/removable: a prosthesis affixed with screws but removable by the patient; fixed-detachable.

Fixture: *See*: ROOT-FORM IMPLANT.

Fixture cover: healing screw.

Flapless implant surgery: implant placement technique whereby neither soft tissue flaps are raised nor a circular piece of tissue is removed.

Flipper: claspless interim all-acrylic denture.

Food and Drug Administration (FDA): a U.S. Department of Health and Human Services agency responsible for assuring the safety, efficacy and security of human and veterinary drugs, biological products, medical devices, U.S. food supply, cosmetics, and products that emit radiation, through testing and regulation.

Force: influence acting on a body and tending to produce or alter motion, and tending to deform the surface of a stable body.

Fossa: anatomic pit or depression.

Fracture: break, rupture, or tear; failure caused by crack growth.

Framework: a reference to the structure of a prosthetic reconstruction; alternatively, the armature or skeleton of a prosthesis.

Free gingiva: keratinized gum surrounding but not attached to the teeth.

Free gingival margin: refers to that distance which is the most coronal portion of the gum tissues surrounding the dental cervix.

Free soft tissue autograft: *See*: GINGIVAL GRAFT.

Free-standing implant: an implant not splinted to adjacent teeth or implants.

Freeze-dried bone allograft (FDBA): refers to bone harvested from donor cadavers, and then washed, immersed in ethanol, frozen in nitrogen, freeze-dried and ground to particles. Particles range in size from 250 to 750 microns. This substance acts primarily osteoconductively as inductive proteins, often found in only minute quantities; the substance's arc is only released after the resorption of the mineral.

Freeze-drying: a dehydration process used to preserve tissue that allows the frozen water in the material to sublime directly from the solid phase to gas.

Frenulum: small fold of integument or mucous membrane checking, limiting, or curbing movements of an organ or part.

Friction-fit: refers to the retention state of an implant at the time of insertion, resulting from slight compression of the implant body walls in the osteotomy. This term also applies to components retained to an implant by friction. *See*: PRESS-FIT.

Fulcrum: a prop or support upon which a lever turns.

Full thickness graft: a graft section of epithelium removed for distant or adjacent repair.

Functional loading: *See*: OCCLUSAL LOADING.

Functional occlusion: contact of teeth providing the highest efficiency in the centric position and during all excursive movements of the jaw essential to mastication without producing trauma.

G

Galvanism: refers to the electropotential difference of dissimilar metals occurring in dental metallurgy in the presence of an electrolyte (such as saliva).

GBR: *Acronym*: Guided bone regeneration.

Genial tubercles: refers to mental spines, small round elevations (usually two pairs) which are clustered around the midline on the lingual surface of the lower portion of the mandibular symphysis; tubercles serve as attachments for the genioglossus and geniohyoid muscles; these tubercles serve as critical landmarks for the subperiosteal implant.

Genioplasty: the use of surgery to alter the chin.

Gingiva: part of the masticatory mucosa covering the alveolar process, surrounding the cervical portion of teeth, and consisting of an epithelial layer and an underlying connective tissue layer (lamina propria).

Gingivae: gum tissues.

Gingival crevice: the space located between the marginal gingivae and a tooth or implant.

Gingival crevicular fluid: fluid originating in the gingival connective tissue that seeps through the sulcular and junctional epithelium, containing sticky plasma proteins which improve adhesions of the epithelial attachment, and have antimicrobial and antibody properties. Flow increases in the presence of inflammation.

Gingival graft: *Syn*: Free soft tissue autograft; surgical procedure to establish adequate keratinized soft tissue around a tooth or an implant or to increase the quantity of soft tissue of an edentulous ridge.

Gingival recession: the apical migration of the marginal gingiva, resulting in exposure of the root surface of the tooth, causing hypersensitivity. One of the main causes of gingival recession is abnormal tooth positioning or trauma.

Glossoplasty: surgical alteration of the tongue.

Glucocorticoid: hormones that affects the metabolism of carbohydrates, fats and proteins made in the adrenal gland and chemically classified as steroids. They act as immuno-suppressants to prevent acute transplant rejection and the graft-versus-host disease. Effective in treating oral lesions.

Glycoprotein: a protein containing one or more covalently linked carbohydrates, plus a protein. Glycoproteins play essential roles in the body such as acting as key molecules in the immune system.

Glycosaminoglycan: (mucopolysaccharide) a binding membrane protein, an important component of connective tissues.

Gnathic: pertaining to the jaw.

Gold cylinder: *See*: PREFABRICATED CYLINDER.

Graft: material used to replace a body's defect; a substance inserted into another substance and intended to become an integral part of the latter. In the case of bone grafts, either artificial or synthetic bone, this graft is usually for the purpose of increasing its strength and/or dimension.

Grafting material: a substance (natural or synthetic) used to repair a tissue defect or deficiency.

Grinding in: a reference to the correction of occlusion.

Grit blasting: delivery of a high velocity stream of abrasive particles propelled by compressed air to an implant surface, to increase its surface area.

Groove: a long, thin depression.

Growth factor: any highly specific protein that is used to stimulate the division and differentiation of cells.

Guide: *See*: RADIOGRAPHIC TEMPLATE, STEREOLITHOGRAPHIC GUIDE, SURGICAL GUIDE.

Guided bone regeneration (GBR): bone regenerative technique using physical means (e.g., membranes) to seal an anatomic site for bone regeneration. The goal of GBR is to direct bone formation and to prevent other tissues (e.g., connective tissue) from interfering with osteogenesis.

Guided tissue regeneration: a procedure designed to direct epithelial and supporting soft tissue restoration and to inhibit epithelial invagination by the use of synthetic membranes.

Guide drill: round drill used to mark an osteotomy site by making an initial entry into cortical bone.

Guide pin: 1. device placed within an osteotomy to determine the location and angulation of the site relative to adjacent teeth, implants, or other landmarks. 2. extended occlusal or abutment screws used during prosthesis fabrication in the laboratory.

Gustation: the sense of taste.

HA: *Acronym*: Hydroxyapatite.

Hadar bar: *See*: DOLDER BAR.

Harvest: gathering or collecting hard or soft tissue for grafting.

Haversian canal: freely anastomosing channels within cortical bone; the channels contain blood and lymph vessels and are surrounded by concentric lamellae of bone.

Healing: regeneration or repair of injured, lost, or surgically treated tissue, occurring by first (primary) intention or by second (secondary) intention.

Healing abutment: *Syn*: Healing collar, permucosal extension, second-stage permucosal abutment, Temporary healing cuff; an abutment connecting to the implant and protruding through the soft tissue. Temporary cuff used after uncovering to facilitate soft tissue healing in the permucosal areas.

Healing by first (primary) intention: *Syn*: Primary closure; wound healing involving the close re-approximation of edges; minimal granulation tissue and scar formation after union.

Healing by second (secondary) intention: *Syn*: Secondary closure; wound healing wound where a gap is left between edges; granulation tissue formation from the base and the sides remains after union. A large amount of epithelial migration, collagen deposition, contraction, and remodeling during healing is required.

Healing cap: *See*: HYGIENE CAP.

Healing collar: *See*: HEALING ABUTMENT.

Healing period: *Syn*: Healing phase; time allocated for healing following a surgery, after which the next procedure is performed at the same site.

Healing phase: *See*: HEALING PERIOD.

Healing screw: refers to the final intra-implant screw placed after first-stage surgery. *See*: COVER SCREW.

Hematopoietic stem cell: progenitor cells from which every lineage including red blood cells, platelets, and a variety of lymphoid and myeloid cells in the body are generated. HSCs are able to generate some of the most important lymphoid cells and myeloid cells including natural killer (NK) cells, T cells, and B cells, granulocytes, monocytes, macrophages, microglial cells, and dendritic cells. HSCs can generate these for many years.

Hemidesmosome: microscope structures which serve as cementing media at the surfaces of epithelial cells; their combinations are called desmosomes when they serve two such adjacent cells.

Hemi-maxillectomy: surgical removal of one portion of the upper jaw, including the premaxilla, maxilla or hard palate.

Hemisection: process of dividing or cutting a tooth or structure into two parts.

Hemocytoblasts: *See*: STEM CELLS.

Hemorrhage: internal or external excessive bleeding.

Hemostasis: the physiologic process of halting bleeding involving three basic mechanisms: vasoconstriction serotonin, ADP and Thromboxane A_2, and finally, coagulation. Also may refer to the process of manually clamping a blood vessel with hemostatic clamps during surgery.

Heterogeneous graft: *See*: XENOGRAFT.

Heterograft: tissue taken from one species and placed into another. *See*: XENOGRAFT.

Hex: a hexagonally-shaped interface connection.

Hex-lock: a six-sided screwdriver or matching screw.

Hexed: component or implant with a hexagonal connection interface.

High lip line: condition in which gingival tissue and crown margins are revealed during smiling.

High-water prosthesis: *See*: HYBRID PROSTHESIS.

Histomorphometry: the study of microstructures; quantitative study of the microscopic tissue organization and structure, especially the computer-assisted analysis of images acquired from a microscope.

Hollow basket implant: a root-form implant with an internal channel that penetrates the implant body at or from its apical aspect.

Homogenous graft: *See*: HOMOGRAFT.

Homograft: *Syn*: Homogenous graft, Homologous graft; a graft transplanted between genetically non-identical individuals of the same species (e.g., a graft taken from one human subject and transplanted into another). *See*: ALLOGRAFT.

Homologous graft: *See*: HOMOGRAFT.

Horseshoe denture: palateless, U-shaped prosthesis.

Host response: local or systemic response of the host organism to the implanted material or device.

Host site: *See*: RECIPIENT SITE.

Hounsfield Unit (HU): x-ray unit attenuation for CT scans to measure bone density; each pixel is assigned a value on a scale (air is —1000, water 0, and compact bone +1000).

HU: *Acronym*: Hounsfield Unit.

Hybrid denture: partial or full denture prosthesis affixed with screws to a mesostructure bar.

Hybrid implant: endosseous, root-form implant consisting of different surface textures at different levels.

Hybrid prosthesis: *Syn*: High-water prosthesis (using long standard abutments with several millimeters of space between the prosthesis and the mucosa of the edentulous ridge); screw-retained, metal-resin, implant-supported, fixed complete denture; implies a combination of a metal framework with a complete denture (i.e., prefabricated resin teeth and heat polymerized resin). *See*: HYBRID DENTURE.

Hydroxyapatite (HA), $Ca_{10}(PO_4)_6(OH)_2$: general term for calcium hydroxylapatite; the primary inorganic and natural component of bone; used as an alloplast and to coat some implant surfaces. *See*: ALLOPLAST.

Hydroxyapatite ceramic: dense, relatively nonresorbable ceramic that displays a highly attractive generic profile featuring a lack of local or systemic reactivity when implanted into bone (pentahydroxyapatite).

Hydroxylapatite: *See*: HYDROXYAPATITE.

Hygiene cap: *Syn*: Comfort cap, Healing cap, Sealing screw; component which is inserted over a prosthetic abutment. The cap's function is to prevent debris and calculus from invading the internal portion of the abutment (between prosthetic appointments).

Hyperbaric oxygenation: administering oxygen under greater than normal pressures, used for therapeutic purposes in the treatment of anaerobic infections (or in areas of ischemia, postradiation.

Hyperbaric oxygen therapy: treatment modality where a patient is placed in a pressurized chamber (hyperbaric chamber), allowing for delivery of oxygen in high concentrations, sometimes used before implant therapy for patients who have undergone radiation therapy in the head and neck areas, thus reducing the risks of osteoradionecrosis.

Hyperesthesia: a reference to abnormally increased sensitivity of skin, mucosa, or an organ of special sense.

Hyperocclusion: Premature tooth contact during mouth closure such as grinding and clenching your teeth which causes a great deal of dental trauma.

Hyperparathyroidism: a chronic disorder of the parathyroid glands involving oversecretion of parathyroid hormone which results in increased bone resorption and increased calcium absorption in the intestines. Main cause of renal failure.

Hyperplasia: abnormal multiplication or increase in the number of normal tissue cells; excessive enlargement of a tissue or structure due to cell number increase.

Hyperplastic tissue: a reference to the enlargement of tissue secondary to a proliferation of normal cells.

Hyperpneumatized sinus: sinus with increased air space. *See*: PNEUMATIZED MAXILLARY SINUS.

Hypertension: commonly known as high blood pressure, a chronic condition where the blood pressure is excessively high.

Hypertrophy: a reference to the increase in tissue bulk beyond normal limits, caused by an increase in size, but not number, of cellular elements.

Hypogeusia: diminished tasting ability.

Hypoplasia: development that is defective or incomplete.

Iatrogenic: a result caused by the activity of the doctor.

Idiopathic: of unknown origin.

IGF: *Acronym*: Insulin-like growth factors.

Iliac crest: superior part of the ilium used as a grafting source of autogenous bone. *See*: ILIAC GRAFT.

Iliac graft: a bone graft which is harvested from the iliac bone's crest; such bone can be removed from the anterior iliac crest posteriorly to the anterosuperior iliac spine or to the posterior ilium. Additionally, this graft may be cancellous, cortical, or cortico-cancellous.

Ilium: the uppermost of the three bones that make up the innominate bone, (or hip bone, the crest of which is a source of bone for mandibular and chin reconstruction and enhancement in dentistry.

Immediate denture: a prosthesis designed for insertion directly after teeth removal.

Immediate functional loading: *See*: IMMEDIATE OCCLUSAL LOADING.

Immediate implant placement: placement of an implant into the extraction socket at the time of tooth extraction.

Immediate loading: *See*: IMMEDIATE OCCLUSAL LOADING, IMMEDIATE NONOCCLUSAL LOADING; the placement into function of newly inserted implants.

Immediate nonfunctional loading: *See*: IMMEDIATE NONOCCLUSAL LOADING.

Immediate nonocclusal loading: a clinical protocol for placing an implant in a partially edentulous arch (at the same clinical visit) with a fixed or removable restoration not in occlusal contact with the opposing dentition. *See*: NONOCCLUSAL LOADING.

Immediate occlusal loading: a clinical protocol for the placement and application of force on implants (at the same clinical visit) with a fixed or removable restoration in occlusal contact with the opposing dentition. *See*: OCCLUSAL LOADING.

Immediate placement: *See*: IMMEDIATE IMPLANT PLACEMENT.

Immediate provisionalization: clinical protocol for placing an interim prosthesis with or without occlusal contact with the opposing dentition, at the same clinical visit of implant placement. *See*: IMMEDIATE NONOCCLUSAL LOADING, IMMEDIATE OCCLUSAL LOADING.

Immediate restoration: *See*: IMMEDIATE PROVISIONALIZATION.

Immediate temporization: *See*: IMMEDIATE PROVISIONALIZATION.

Immunologic response: a bodily defense in the form of a reaction that recognizes an invading substance (an antigen: such as a virus or fungus or bacteria or transplanted organ) and produces antibodies specific against that antigen.

Implant (noun): device designed for surgical insertion into the body, including an alloplastic material or device that is surgically placed into the oral tissue, for anchorage, functional, therapeutic, and/or esthetic purposes.

Implant (verb): the surgical act of placing a device into the body.

Implant abutment: *See*: ABUTMENT.

Implant-abutment junction: *Syn*: Microgap; margin of connection between the implant's coronal aspect and the prosthetic abutment or restoration.

Implant anchorage: support for orthodontic tooth movement or arch expansion provided by an implant.

Implant-assisted prosthesis: any prosthesis completely or partly supported by an implant or implants. *See*: IMPLANT-

IMPLANT HEAD

SUPPORTED PROSTHESIS, IMPLANT-TISSUE-SUPPORTED PROSTHESIS; CEMENT-RETAINED, FIXED PROSTHESIS, HYBRID PROSTHESIS, REMOVABLE PROSTHESIS, SCREW-RETAINED.

Implant attachment: *See*: ATTACHMENT.

Implant body: *Syn*: Implant shaft; the portion of a root-form implant available for bone-to-implant contact; the infrastructure.

Implant collar: the smooth part that can be found just apical to the edge of the platform or the implant-abutment junction, the root-form implants has a collar.

Implant connecting bar: a cast or welded bar which connects one implant to another.

Implant crown: a casting placed over an implant abutment, which is designed to assume the role of a natural crown.

Implant dentistry: type of dentistry concerned with the diagnosis, design, and insertion of implant devices and implant restorations to provide increases function, comfort, and aesthetics for the edentulous or partially edentulous patient. *Syn*: Oral implantology.

Implant denture: a denture receiving stability and retention from a dental implant.

Implant exposure: a postoperative condition whereby an implant is not completely covered by soft tissue due to an bursting open or splitting along sutured lines.

Implant fixture: *See*: IMPLANT.

Implant head: the segment of the subperiosteal or blade implant above the neck, used to connect to the prosthetic reconstruction. *Syn*: Abutment.

Implant infrastructure: that segment of an implant of any type designed to achieve retention. *See*: IMPLANT BODY.

Implant integration: a reference to tissue-to-implant contact.

Implant interface: a reference to that site created by an implant and its adjacent supporting tissues; area of contact between tissues (for example, bone, connective tissue) and the implant surface.

Implant length: data for implants involving the straight-line measurement from the implant crown surface to the end tip of the implant screw.

Implant level impression: the impression of the implant platform that uses an implant impression coping. *See*: ABUTMENT LEVEL IMPRESSION.

Implant loading: placement of prosthetic devices so that an implant can be brought into function.

Implant micromovement: microscopic movement of a dental implant amidst soft tissue. Primary stability of dental implants is critical for their osseointegration.

Implant mount: device used to transfer an implant to the prepared surgical site.

Implant neck: *Syn*: Cervix. 1. Root-form implant: the most coronal aspect of an implant. 2. Subperiosteal or Blade implant: the transmucosal segment which connects the implant to the head or abutment.

Implantology: the art and science of diagnosis, treatment, maintenance, and problem management of implant-dentistry.

Implant periapical lesion: radiolucency localized at the apex of a root-form implant, either asymptomatic or symptomatic (acute), which may include fistula with purulent exudate and/or pain on palpation.

Implant prosthesis: a denture which is supported wholly or partly by implants. Any (fixed, removable, or maxillofacial) prosthesis using dental implants for retention, support, and stability.

Implant prosthodontics: implant dentistry concerned with the diagnosis, presurgical planning, construction, and placement of fixed or removable prostheses on any dental implant device; concerns the construction and placement of fixed or removable prostheses on any implant device.

Implant-retained prosthesis: any prosthesis completely or partly supported by an implant or implants. *See*: IMPLANT-CEMENT-RETAINED, FIXED PROSTHESIS, HYBRID PROSTHESIS, REMOVABLE PROSTHESIS, SCREW-RETAINED.

Implant shaft: *See*: IMPLANT BODY.

Implant site: the area in the alveolar ridge where the implant is to be inserted in restorative surgery.

Implant soft tissue management: use of special techniques during the pre-implant phase, and during implant integration to maintain the periodontal health and restorative aspects of soft tissue in and after implant surgery.

Implant splinting: connection of restorative components with a bar or an overdenture typically between implant abutments and natural teeth to enhance strength.

Implant stability: the variables in movement of an implant within the surrounding bone after testing. Implant stability is depedent to local bone density and subject to changes due to bone remodeling.

Implant stability quotient (ISQ): the measure of implant stability (from 1 to 100, 100 being the highest degree of stability) obtained from resonance frequency analysis.

Implant substructure: *See*: INFRASTRUCTURE.

Implant success: implant status based on predetermined success criteria. *See*: IMPLANT SURVIVAL.

Implant superstructure: prosthesis permitted to rest on implants, on a mesostructure bar, or on natural tissue and implants.

Implant-supported prosthesis: a restoration whose entire support is from dental implants. This type of restoration may be fixed or removable, partial or complete arch. *See*: FIXED PROSTHESIS, REMOVABLE PROSTHESIS.

Implant surface: *See*: SURFACE CHARACTERISTICS (IMPLANT).

Implant surgery: portion of implant dentistry that concerns the placement and exposure of implant devices; the area of implant dentistry concerning the placement, surgical repair, and removal of implant devices.

Implant survival: implant longevity within the oral cavity. *See*: IMPLANT SUCCESS.

Implant system: a set of instruments and supplies designed to perform the various steps of implant insertion and prosthetic reconstruction.

Implant thread: *See*: THREAD.

Implant-tissue-supported prosthesis: restoration deriving its support from a combination of intraoral tissues and dental implants, always removable and either partial or complete arch. *See*: FIXED PROSTHESIS, REMOVABLE PROSTHESIS.

Implant try-in: *See*: TRIAL FIT GAUGE.

Impression: a negative likeness (reverse copy) of the surface of an object or anatomic part.

Impression coping: device for registering the position of a dental implant or dental implant abutment in an impression. The coping may be retained in the impression (direct) or may require a transfer from intraoral usage to the impression after the attachment of the corresponding analog (indirect).

Impression tray: special trays made from acrylic or shellac consisting of a body with a handle used to contain a material (e.g., rubber, hydrocolloid, or alginate) to place against the palatal tissues for making a mold of teeth.

Incisive foramen: a critical landmark for implant dentistry, and one of many openings of incisive canals into the incisive fossa, located in the midline on the anterior extreme of the hard palate; it transmits the left (more anterior) and right (more posterior) nasopalatine (Scarpa's; long sphenopalatine) nerves and vessels.

Incisive papilla: soft tissue mound which overlies the incisive foramen and neurovascular bundle, found immediately palatal to the central incisors.

Inclusion criteria: specific characteristics that all participants must have to enter a clinical trial. *See*: EXCLUSION CRITERIA.

Index: mold for recording the relative position of an implant or tooth to its surroundings. *See*: BUCCAL INDEX.

Indirect impression: *See*: CLOSED TRAY IMPRESSION.

Indirect transfer coping: prosthetic device permitting the laboratory technician to restore the case on a cast.

Indurated: hard.

Inferior alveolar artery: *(arteria alveolaris inferio)r* the artery that runs through the mandibular canal to supply the lower teeth.

Inferior alveolar canal: *See*: MANDIBULAR CANAL.

Inferior alveolar nerve: one of the terminal branches of the mandibular nerve, a division of the trigeminal nerve, entering the mandibular canal and branching to the lower teeth, periosteum, and gingiva of the mandible. One branch, the mental nerve, passes through the mental foramen, supplying the skin and mucosa of the lower lip and chin.

Inflammation: a process by which the body's white blood cells and chemicals protect it from infection and foreign substances such as bacteria and viruses by forming a protective wall, accompanied by heat, redness, soreness, pain, itching, and/or swelling.

Informed consent: a process of communication between a patient and oral surgeon that results in the patient's full awareness of risks and benefits of, and subsequent authorization to undergo a specific medical procedure.

Infracture: controlled fracture of: 1. the lateral wall of the maxillary sinus for a window. 2. The floor of the maxillary sinus through an osteotomy prepared in the ridge.

Infraocclusion: below the biting plane.

Infrastructure: framework upon which a denture is processed; implants supporting a prosthetic reconstruction.

Initial stability: *Syn*: Primary stability; degree implant tightness immediately after placement in the prepared osteotomy. Implant initial stability is measured by clinical immobile at placement.

Insertion torque: torque value used to insert an implant into an osteotomy, expressed in Newtons centimeter.

Insulin-like growth factors (IGF): peptides that behave similarly to insulin and stimulate cell proliferation. *See*: PLATELET-RICH PLASMA.

Integration: melding of an implant surface with its supporting tissues.

Interdental bone height: vertical distance from the crest of bone to the height of the interproximal papilla between two teeth or adjacent implants.

Interdental papilla: portion of the free gingiva which occupies the interproximal space confined by adjacent teeth in contact; triangular projections of gingival tissue extending between the teeth. *See*: PAPILLA.

Interdigitation: interlocking of protruding processes (fingers, teeth).

Interface: *See*: IMPLANT INTERFACE.

Interfacial: zone between an implant and adjacent supporting tissue.

Interim endosteal dental implant abutment: temporary abutment to retain an interim prosthesis.

Interimplant distance: horizontal distance between the platforms of two adjacent implants.

Interimplant papilla: soft tissue which occupies the interproximal space confined by adjacent implant-supported fixed partial dentures in contact *See*: PAPILLA.

Interim prosthesis/restoration: *Syn*: Provisional prosthesis/ restoration; denture used during healing or while a final prosthesis is being fabricated. A fixed or removable prosthesis, designed to restore and enhance esthetics, stabilization or function for a limited time; used as a diagnostic tool to mimic the planned definitive prosthesis; may be tissue-born, tooth-supported, implant-supported, or any combination.

Interlock: male-female device used to create a relationship between two prostheses, one of which must be fixed.

Interleukins: a class of proteins that are secreted mostly by macrophages and T lymphocytes and induce growth and differentiation of lymphocytes and hematopoietic stem cells. Linked to periodontal and peri-implanter disease.

Intermediate abutment: tooth or implant located between natural or tooth abutments; a pier abutment.

Internal connection: prosthetic connection interface internal to the implant platform (e.g., hexagon and Morse taper). *See*: EXTERNAL CONNECTION.

Internal hexagon: hexagonal connection interface of the platform of an implant within coronal aspect; prevents rotation of attached components. *See*: EXTERNAL HEXAGON.

Internal irrigation: irrigation during drilling of osteotomies for placement of root-form implants so that cooling solution passes inside the shaft of the drilling bur and is delivered through an exit at the working end. the cooling solution is delivered inside the osteotomy. *See*: EXTERNAL IRRIGATION.

INTRAORAL (INTERNAL) DISTRACTION DEVICE

Internally-threaded: thread pattern within the implant body.

Interocclusal distance: the distance between the occlusal surfaces of opposing teeth of the mandibular and maxillary arches.

Interproximal space (embrasure): area between two adjacent teeth, which may be gingival to (greater embrasure) or incisal to (lesser embrasure) the contact point.

Interpupillary line: imaginary line that connects the centers of the pupils and is helpful for frontal facial symmetry when arranging prosthetics and implants.

Intramembranous ossification: sheet-like connective tissue membranes (not cartilage) with bony tissue. Bones formed in this manner include flat bones of the skull and some of the irregular bones.

Intramucosal insert: alloplastic devices placed into tissue-borne surface of a removable prosthesis to mechanically maintain the mucostatic seal; the insert is generally made of titanium or surgical stainless steel and shaped with a narrow permucosal neck, a wider retentive head, and a broad, flat, denture-attaching base; general utilization: maxillary complete denture or mandibular and maxillary removable partial dentures; also called mucosal insert or subdermal implant. *See*: MUCOSAL INSERT.

Intraoral distraction: procedure in which a device is located completely within the oral cavity for distraction osteogenesis.

Intraoral (internal) distraction device: device located within the oral cavity and used in distraction osteogenesis. The device can be attached to the bone (bone-borne), to the teeth (tooth-borne), or simultaneously to the teeth and bone (hybrid).

Intraosseous: within the bone.

Intraosseous distractor: *See*: ENDOSSEOUS DISTRACTOR.

In vitro: outside the organism or natural system, refers to artificial experimental systems such as cultures or cell-free extracts.

In vivo: within the living organism or natural system.

Irrigation: 1. Technique of using a solution, usually saline, to cool the surgical bur and wash the debris off the flutes. 2. Act of flushing an area with a solution. *See*: EXTERNAL IRRIGATION, INTERNAL IRRIGATION.

Ischemia: loss of tissue blood supply due to pathologic or mechanical obstruction, and which may result in cell death and necrosis. Blood deficiency due to functional constriction or actual obstruction of a blood vessel(s).

Isogeneic graft: *See*: ISOGRAFT.

Isograft: *Syn*: Isogeneic graft, Isologous graft, Syngeneic graft; tissue graft transplanted from one genetically identical individual to another, as in monozygotic twins.

Isologous graft: *See*: ISOGRAFT.

Isometric contraction: muscle tightening with no change in muscle length.

Isotonic contraction: muscle tightening with change in muscle length and constant tension.

Isotropic surface: Surface textures which are randomly distributed so that the surface is identical in all directions. *See*: ANISOTROPIC SURFACE.

J

Jacob Creuzfeldt disease: transmissible degenerative brain disorder technically termed spongiform encephalopathy; symptoms may include forgetfulness, nervousness, trembling hand, unsteady gait, muscle spasms, chronic dementia, balance disorder, and loss of facial expression; can be caused by consumption of "mad cow" meat or squirrel brains.

Jaw: one of two bony structures where teeth are found.

Jig: a dental restoration device in which dowels are employed to locate and register teeth. *See*: ORIENTATION JIG, VERIFICATION JIG.

Joint-separating force: force attempting to disengage screw-joined parts.

Junctional epithelium: epithelium adhering to the surface of implant or tooth at the base of the sulcus; constitutes the coronal part of the biologic width and formed by single or multiple layers of nonkeratinizing cells. The junctional epithelial cells have a basal membrane and hemidesmosomal attachments to the surface of implant or tooth. *See*: EPITHELIAL ATTACHMENT.

K

Kaplan-Meier analysis: statistical method to estimate a population (e.g., implants) survival curve from a sample. Survival over time can be estimated even if patients drop out or are studied for different lengths of time.

Keratin: a protein found in all comified body structures (e.g., hair, nails, teeth, and fixed gingiva).

Keratinized gingiva: portion of the mucosa covered by keratinized epithelium; part of the oral mucosa covering the gingiva and hard palate, extending from the free gingival margin to the mucogingival junction. It consists of the free gingiva and the attached gingiva.

Knife-edge: (knife-edge ridge) a term used to describe a residual ridge's extremely sharp, narrow morphology.

Knoop hardness testing: method of using varying pressures with a diamond stylus to test a material's surface hardness.

L

Labial: pertaining to the lip; in the direction of the lip.

Laboratory analog: *See*: ANALOG.

Lamellar bone: *See*: Bone.

Lamina dura: thin cortical bone plate bone which functions as tooth socket lining.

Lapping tool: instrument used for precise finishing of surfaces; instrument used to remove the uneven surface produced during a lab's casting process of an abutment.

Laser: (Light Amplification by the Stimulated Emission of Radiation) a device that emits a very narrow, highly concentrated beam of light that can be focused on tight areas. Lasers have a variety of uses. They function by pumping photons out of a chamber with mirrors at both ends. Output can be continuous or pulsed.

Laser etching: the use of a laser beam selectively to ablate a material from a surface (e.g., implant).

Laser welding: connecting titanium implants, bars, and so on by using the noninvasive electrons of a machine developed by Arturo Hruska.

Late implant failure: *Syn*: Secondary implant failure; failure of a root-form implant after osseointegration due to or accompanied by peri-implantitis or overload. *See*: EARLY IMPLANT FAILURE.

Latency period: *See*: DISTRACTION OSTEOGENESIS.

Lateral: sideways; to the side.

Lateral window technique: creation of an access to the maxillary sinus through the lateral wall to elevate the Schneiderian membrane for graft placement in the sinus through the prepared opening.

Le Fort osteotomy: a surgery separating the maxilla and the palate from the skull above the roots of the upper teeth. The maxilla is repositioned in its new position with titanium screws and plates. There are three types Le Fort I, II, and III.

Leukocyte: a white blood cell. A blood cell that does not contain hemoglobin. Cells made by bone marrow that help the body fight infection and other diseases.

Life table analysis: Statistical method for describing the survival in a sample (e.g., implants). Survival time is divided into a certain number of intervals, and for each interval, computation can determine the number and proportion of cases that entered the respective interval "alive," the number and proportion of cases that failed in the respective interval (i.e., number of cases that "died"), and the number of cases that were lost or censored in said interval.

Light microscopy: method for viewing specimens via a device offering conventional enlargement.

Linea alba: white line; a reference to the midcrestal scar caused by extractions and secondary healing.

Lingual: pertaining to the tongue; on the side of the tongue.

Lining mucosa: *See*: ALVEOLAR MUCOSA, ORAL MUCOSA.

Lip line: the point or level during smiling where the lip can be found.

Load: a reference to any external mechanical force which is applied to a prosthesis, implant, abutment, tooth, skeletal organ, or tissue.

Loading: a reference the placing of an implant or tooth into functional occlusion; application of a force directly or indirectly to an implant.

Localization film(s): a method use to determine the site of a foreign body by using one or several multi-angle radiographs.

Longitudinal study: observations of the same subjects at two or more different times.

Lute: to attach, cement, affix, join, spot-weld, or solder.

Lyophilization: preferred method of preservation in the medical industry, regularly used to preserve vaccines, pharmaceuticals, blood, plasma, and other fragile substances. Commonly known as "freeze-drying."

Machined surface: *Syn*: Turned surface; an implant surface that has undergone the milling process of a cylindrical titanium rod. Tooled etches on the implant form a machined implant surface. *See*: SURFACE CHARACTERISTICS (IMPLANT), TEXTURED SURFACE.

Macroglossia: enlargement of the tongue.

Macrointerlock: mechanical interlocking between bone and implant macro- irregularities such as threads, holes, pores, grooves, and so on, which have dimensions in the range of 100μm or greater.

Macromotion: excess movement which prevents bone healing and osseointegration, resulting in fibrous tissue encapsulation. *See*: MICROMOTION.

Macrophage: a mononuclear, actively phagocytic cell originating from specific monocytic stem cells in bone marrow, widely distributed throughout the body that vary in morphology and digest cellular debris and pathogens and stimulate lymphocytes and other immune cells to respond to the pathogen. Large, long-lived cells with nearly round nuclei and abundant endocytic vacuoles, endosomes, lysosomes, and phagolysosomes.

Magnet: device used for retention of overdentures.

Magnetic resonance imaging (MRI): a diagnostic radiologic modality, using nuclear magnetic resonance technology in which the magnetic nuclei (especially protons) of a patient absorb energy from radiofrequency pulses, and emit radiofrequency signals then converted into sets of high-quality, 3-dimensional images of their point sources, without use of x-rays or radioactive tracers.

Maintenance: procedures at selected time intervals to maintain prosthetic reconstruction and periodontal and peri-implant health.

Malleable: material capable of enlargement or shaping by pressure rollers or a mallet.

Malpositioned implant: dental implants that are ill-fitting or faulty, inserted incorrectly in the alveolar ridge and unusable.

Malpractice litigation: a part of tort law, where negligence is the predominant theory of liability. Medical malpractice is improper, illegal, or negligent professional activity or treatment by a medical practitioner. A person who alleges medical malpractice must prove four elements: (1) a duty of care was owed by the physician; (2) the physician violated the applicable standard of care; (3) the person suffered a compensable injury; and (4) the injury was caused in fact and proximately caused by the substandard conduct. The plaintiff has the burden of proof and the critical element is "standard of care."

Mandible: the bone of the lower jaw consisting of a "body" which is a curved, horizontal portion and the "rami" which are two perpendicular portions uniting the ends of the body nearly at right angles. It is the largest and strongest bone of the face.

Mandibular block graft: intraoral source of autogenous block graft taken from the ramus buccal shelf or the mandibular symphysis, and surgically attached to a prepared site to enhance bone volume and density, allowing for placement of implants to facilitate stress distribution.

Mandibular canal: *Syn*: Inferior alveolar canal; canal within the mandible holding the inferior alveolar nerve and vessels. The posterior opening is the mandibular foramen, and anterior opening is the mental foramen.

Mandibular flexure: deformation in the body of the mandible caused by contraction of the pterygoid muscles during opening and protrusion.

Mandibular foramen: opening into the mandibular canal on the medial surface of the ramus giving passage to the inferior alveolar nerve, artery, and vein.

Mandibular nerve: the third division of the trigeminal nerve, leaving the skull through the foramen ovale and providing motor innervation to the muscles of mastication and to the

M

tensor tympani, the anterior belly of the digastric, and the mylohyoid muscles; this nerve also provides general sensory innervation to the teeth, gingivae, the mucosa of the cheek, floor of the mouth, the epithelium of the anterior two thirds of the tongue, the meninges, and the skin of the lower portion of the face.

Mandibular staple implant: *Syn*: Transmandibular implant; also called a bone plate; a form of a transosseous implant; a plate is placed at the inferior border and a series of retentive pins is placed partially into the inferior border, with two continuous screws placed transcortically and penetrating the mouth in the canine areas for abutments.

Mandrel: device used in a handpiece, permitting the mounting of a stone or disc for grinding or finishing a restoration.

Marginal peri-implant area: the mucosal peri-implant tissues and marginal bone.

Master cast: the final model representing the exact positioning of the abutments for fabrication of a prosthesis.

Masticate: chew.

Masticatory mucosa: keratinized and attached oral mucosa of gingiva and hard palate. *See*: ORAL MUCOSA.

Matrix: intricate network of natural or synthetic fibers aiding the reinforcement and development of tissues by supplying a scaffold for cells to grow, migrate, and proliferate.

Maxillary antroplasty: *See*: SINUS GRAFT.

Maxillary antrum: *See*: MAXILLARY SINUS.

Maxillary artery: the larger of the two terminal branches of the external carotid artery which starts behind the neck of the mandible and supplies the face with blood.

Maxillary sinus: *Syn*: Antrum of Highmore, Maxillary antrum; bilateral cavities in the maxillary bone located above the dentition, lateral to the nose, inferior to the orbits, and lined with respiratory epithelium. Air cavity within the maxilla, lined by the Schneiderian membrane, consisting of a pseudo-stratified ciliated columnar epithelium. The maxillary sinus lies superior to the roots of premolars and molars, generally extending from the canine or premolar region posterior to the molar or tuberosity region. The cavity is pyramidal, with thin, bony walls corresponding to the orbital, alveolar (floor), facial, and infra-temporal aspects of the maxilla. The apex extends into the zygomatic process, and its base is medial, forming the lateral wall of the nasal cavity. The sinus communicates with the nasal cavity through an opening (ostium) in the middle meatus. The floor of the maxillary sinus is formed by the maxillary alveolar process and by the hard palate. The floor of the maxillary sinus has recesses and depressions in the premolar and molar regions. Each of the sinuses usually has a volume of about 15 ml. *See*: ALVEOLAR RECESS, SEPTUM (MAXILLARY SINUS).

Maxillary sinusitis: inflammation of the maxillary sinuses which produces pain over the cheeks just below the eyes, a toothache, and headache. It may or may not be as a result of infection, from bacterial, fungal, viral, allergic, or autoimmune issues.

Maxillary sinus membrane: thin mucous membrane lining the sinus cavity.

Maxillary sinus pneumatization: air cells or cavities in tissue, which usually fluid-filled at birth. The growth of these sinuses is biphasic with growth during years 0-3 and 7-12. During the later phase pneumatization spreads more inferiorly as permanent teeth take their place.

Maxillary tuberosity: most distal structure of the maxillary alveolar ridge; bulbous in configuration, the tuberosity is usually located behind the third molars.

Maxillofacial prosthesis: an artificial replacement of the jaw bone.

Maxillofacial prosthetics: a branch of dentistry that deals with congenital and acquired defects of the head and neck. Maxillofacial prosthetics integrates parts of multiple disciplines including head and neck oncology, congenital malformation, plastic surgery, speech, and other related disciplines.

Mean (arithmetic): measure of central tendency, calculated by adding all the individual values in the group and dividing by the number of group values.

Mechanical failure: implant (or abutment or restorative component or material) fracture or deformation.

Mechanicoreceptor: nerve endings that respond to mechanical stimuli.

Median: measure of central tendency; the middle score in a distribution or set of ranked scores. The median is computed as the average of the two middle values when the number of values in the sample is even.

Medical-grade calcium sulfate: a ceramic filling material in bone cavities which is resorbable and has been used to fill cavities for more than 100 years. The main sources of calcium sulfate are naturally-occurring gypsum.

Medullary: pertaining to the bone marrow.

Medullary bone: *See*: BONE.

Membrane: thin layer of tissue or material (usually a lining). *See*: BARRIER MEMBRANE, SCHNEIDERIAN MEMBRANE.

Mental foramen: anterior opening of the mandibular canal on the lateral aspect of the body of the mandible; the foramen gives passage to the mental artery and nerve.

Mental nerve: a branch of the inferior alveolar nerve, arising in the mandibular canal and passing through the mental foramen; the mental nerve provides sensation to the chin and lower lip.

Mensenchymal cell: also known as the mesenchymal stem cell or MSC that contributes to regeneration of mesenchymal tissues such as bone, cartilage, muscle, ligament, and tendons. The best source for MSC is bone marrow. Known to stimulate growth of hemopoietic cells within bone marrow.

Mesostructure: that part of a construction which joins the implant complex (infrastructure) to the superstructure.

M

Meta-analysis: quantitative method for combining the results of independent studies which meet specified protocol criteria (usually drawn from the published literature) and synthesize summaries and conclusions that may be used to evaluate therapeutic effectiveness and to plan new studies.

Metal: strong, relatively ductile substance providing electropositive ions to a corrosive environment; can be highly polished.

Metal encapsulator: *See*: METAL HOUSING.

Metal housing: *Syn*: Metal encapsulator; part of an attachment mechanism incorporated in a removable prosthesis; the interchangeable plastic retentive component which is inserted in the metal housing and replaced when necessary.

Metal tap: *See*: TAP.

Methylmethacrylate: an organic compound with the formula $CH_2=C(CH_3)CO_2CH_3$ which is used in the production in the production of the transparent plastic polymethyl methacrylate (PMMA) also known as resin.

Metronidazole: (Flagyl) an antibiotic that fights bacteria in your body mainly in the treatment of infections caused by susceptible organisms, and used to treat periodontitis and peri-implantitis.

Microfracture: minuscule crack in solid material caused either by stress or (manufacturing) flaw that could lead to structural failure.

Microgap: space (usually measured in microns) between two structures or devices. *See*: IMPLANT-ABUTMENT JUNCTION.

Microglossia: small tongue.

Micrognathia: small jaw.

Microinterlock: fixation from mechanical interlocking of bone to micro-irregularities at the implant surface (e.g., machined surfaces, texture from grit blasting, coating, ion bombardment, or irregularities from plasma spraying, and so on); the interlocking has dimensions in the range of microns.

Microlock: very small device designed to securely and reliably affix a prosthesis.

Micromotion: movement which does not stop bone ingrowth of an implant, resulting in direct bone anchorage of the implant (osseointegration). *See*: MACROMOTION.

Microstomia: small oral orifice.

Microtia: small ear.

Midcrestal incision: incision in the middle of the alveolar crest. *See*: CRESTAL INCISION, MUCOBUCCAL FOLD INCISION.

Millipore filter: a trade name for filters made of a meshwork of cellulose acetate or nitrate with a defined pore size. They can be autoclaved and are used for filtering out microorganisms. They are about 150m thick.

Mini-implant: implant that is smaller than standard dental rootform implant, cheaper, and allows for immediate loading. They are 1.8 mm in diameter and come in 4 lengths from which to choose, depending on the amount of bone available to retain the implant, as well as an assessment of the density of the bone. Mini implants are used for supporting crowns in situations in which there is not enough room for a standard implant.

Mobile: loose or movable.

Mode: score or value occurring most frequently in a distribution.

Modeling (bone): independent sites of formation and resorption resulting in shape or size change of bone. Modeling occurs during growth and healing.

Modulus of elasticity: stress-over-strain ratio when deformation is elastic. A measure of material stiffness or flexibility. Stiff material has a high modulus of elasticity while flexible material has a low modulus (also called Young's modulus). *See*: ELASTICITY.

Monocortical: a specimen or bone with a single external dense covering.

Monocyte: a large white blood cell formed in bone marrow and spleen which removes dead or damaged tissues, destroys cancer cells, and regulates immunity against foreign substances.

Monomer: chemical (usually liquid) which can undergo polymerization, either by itself or with a compatible powder.

Morse taper connection: an internal connection interface which consists of a converging circular surface forming a mechanical locking friction-fit. *Syn*: Cold weld.

Moulage: a facial moulage; a procedure used to record the contours of the face by making a molding (moulage) and model of the face.

Mucobuccal fold: cul-de-sac formed by the mucous membrane when turning from the upper or lower gingivae to the cheek.

Mucobuccal fold incision: *Syn*: Vestibular incision; an incision made in the mucobuccal fold. *See*: CRESTAL INCISION, MIDCRESTAL INCISION.

Mucocele: an oral mucous retention cyst, from a ruptured salivary gland duct usually caused by local trauma, commonly found in children and young adults.

Mucogingival junction: demarcation which occurs between the masticatory mucosa and the alveolar mucosa. Border which exists between fixed and areolar gingivae.

Mucogingival surgery: surgical procedures to augment the band of soft-tissue defects around the teeth used in periodontics. One of which is to create a flap of gingival tissue repositioned apically to maintain a functionally adequate zone of attached gingiva.

Mucoperiosteal flap: a full-thickness flap of mucosal tissue, including the periosteum, gingival, and alveolar mucosa, reflected from a bone.

Mucoperiosteum: layer of mucosa, connective tissue, and periosteum covering bone in the oral cavity, sometimes giving rise to muscle attachments.

Mucosa: a membrane composed of epithelium and lamina propria lining the oral cavity and other organs and cavities of the body; also called mucous membrane. The epithelial lining of body cavities, consisting of a mucous membrane and opening to the outside. *See*: ORAL MUCOSA.

Mucosal implant: *See*: MUCOSAL INSERT.

Mucosal insert: *Syn*: Button implant, Epithelial implant, Intramucosal insert, Mucosal implant; a mushroom-shaped device which is fastened to the tissue surface of a removable denture and which fits within a prepared gingival receptor site and, in conjunction with other, multiple inserts, enhances denture retention and stability.

Mucosal peri-implant tissues: soft tissues (epithelium and connective) around an implant.

Mucositis: inflammation of the mucosa. *See*: PERI-IMPLANT MUCOSITIS.

Multicenter study: clinical trial conducted on a single protocol but at more than one research center and by more than one investigator.

Muscle mold: the shaping of material by manipulation or action of the tissues adjacent to the impression's borders; also called border mold.

Mylohyoid ridge: oblique ridge on the lingual surface of the mandible, extending from the level of the roots of the last molar as a bony attachment for the mylohyoid muscles which form the floor of the mouth; the ridge determines the lingual boundary of the mandibular subperiosteal implant.

Myositis: muscle inflammation.

N

Nasal spine: median, sharp process which is formed by the forward prolongation of two maxillae at the lower margin of the anterior aperture of the nose; used to support a maxillary subperiosteal implant.

Nasopalatine nerve: branch of the pterygopalatine ganglion passing through the sphenopalatine foramen, crossing to and then down the nasal septum and through the incisive foramen; this nerve supplies the mucous membrane of the anterior hard palate.

Navigation: *See*: COMPUTER-AIDED NAVIGATION.

Ncm: *Acronym*: Newton centimeter.

Nd:YAG laser: a crystal that is used as a medium for solid-state lasers. Nd:YAG lasers are used for soft tissue surgeries in the oral cavity, such as gingivectomy, periodontal sulcular debridement, frenectomy, and coagulation of graft donor sites.

Necrosis: death of cells or tissue, caused by loss of blood supply, by bacterial toxins, or by physical and chemical agents.

Nerve lateralization: *See*: NERVE REPOSITIONING.

Nerve repositioning: *Syn*: Nerve lateralization, Nerve transpositioning; surgical procedure during which the course of the inferior alveolar nerve is redirected so as to increase the clinician's ability to place longer implants in a mandible which has experienced extensive resorption of the posterior ridge.

Nerve transpositioning: *See*: NERVE REPOSITIONING.

N

Neuralgia: pain experienced along a sensory nerve pathway.

Neuritis: inflammation of a nerve.

Neurovascular bundle: a term applied to the body's nerves, arteries, veins, and lymphatics lying between the innermost and the inner intercostal muscles.

Neuropathy: any functional disturbance or change to a nerve.

Newton centimeter: (Ncm) Unit of rotational torque.

Nidus: a place or central point from which organisms emanate

Nightguard: *See*: OCCLUSAL GUARD.

Noble metals: elements resistant to oxidation, corrosion, and tarnishing during heating operations in a saline environment.

Nonabsorbable: description of a material which does not degrade in vivo over time. *See*: NONRESORBABLE.

Nonangled abutment: *See*: NONANGULATED ABUTMENT

Nonangulated abutment: *Syn*: Nonangled abutment, Straight abutment; abutment with a body parallel to the long axis of the implant. *See*: ANGULATED ABUTMENT.

Nonaxial loading: the application of forces off the implant long-axis. *See*: AXIAL LOADING.

Nonfunctional loading: *See*: NONOCCLUSAL LOADING.

Nonhexed: implant component or an implant without a hexagonal connection interface.

Nonlamellar bone: *See*: BONE.

Nonocclusal loading: restoration not in occlusal contact with the opposing dentition in maximal intercuspal position or in excursions, though there may be restoration contact with the cheeks, tongue, lips, and food. *See*: OCCLUSAL LOADING.

Nonresorbable: description of material which does not degrade over time or which show relatively limited in vivo degradation. *See*: NONABSORBABLE.

Nonsubmergible: not buried.

Nonsubmergible implant: *See*: ONE-STAGE IMPLANT.

Nonthreaded implant: endosseous, root-form implant with no threads, may be parallel-sided (i.e., cylindrical) or tapered.

O

Obtundent: material used to obturate or seal.

Obturator: prosthesis designed to seal an acquired or congenital defect.

Occlude: to close.

Occlusal dysesthesia: refers to unusual perceptions of the bite.

Occlusal equilibration: balance between opposing elements of the masticatory apparatus.

Occlusal guard: removable appliance designed to minimize effects of bruxism and other occlusal habits which may damage dental implants, dentition, and prosthetic reconstruction.

O

Occlusal loading: refers the restoration's occlusal contact with the opposing dentition in maximal intercuspal position and/or excursions. *See*: NONOCCLUSAL LOADING.

Occlusal overload: *See*: OVERLOAD.

Occlusal table: the masticating surfaces grinding surfaces of the bicuspid and molar teeth, and other posterior teeth.

Occlusion: the manner in which the maxillary (upper) and mandibular (lower) teeth come together when they approach each other, as occurs during chewing, or when the mouth is closed.

Occlusive membrane: *See*: BARRIER MEMBRANE.

Odontalgia: toothache.

Oligodontia: fewer than the normal complement of teeth.

One-part implant: *Syn*: One-piece implant; implant without a surface joint exposed to tissues since the endosseous and transmucosal portions consist of a single unit. *See*: TWO-PART IMPLANT.

One-piece abutment: abutment connecting to the implant without an additional screw, retained by cement, friction (press-fit), or screw threads. *See*: TWO-PIECE ABUTMENT.

One-piece implant: *See*: ONE-PART IMPLANT.

One-screw test: a method for checking the fit of a multiple-unit screw-retained restoration. A single screw is placed in the terminal abutment, and evaluation is made on the opposite side. Fit is inaccurate when a clinical or radiological examination determines that the framework rises or has a ledge.

One-stage implant: *Syn*: Nonsubmergible implant, Single-stage implant; endosseous implant designed with a transmucosal coronal portion (one-piece implant with no microgap) and placed in a one-stage surgery protocol. *See*: TWO-STAGE IMPLANT.

One-stage implant placement: single surgical procedure where the site is prepared, implant placed, and there is no need for second surgical procedure.

One-stage surgery: placing an endosseous root-form implant in the bone and leaving it in contact with the oral environment during the healing process, eliminating a second surgical procedure. *See*: TWO-STAGE SURGERY.

Onlay graft: an autogenous bone or bone replacement graft or both placed on or over bone to increase length or width or both.

Open-ended wrench: Instrument for applying torque during removal of an implant mount.

Open tray impression: *Syn*: Direct impression; technique using an impression coping with retentive features around which a rigid elastic impression material is injected. The impression coping is first unthreaded through an opening on the occlusal surface of the tray before removal. *See*: CLOSED TRAY IMPRESSION.

Oral flora: organisms in the mouth.

Oral implant: biomaterial or device made of one or more biomaterials, biologic or alloplastic, surgically inserted into soft or hard tissues for functional or cosmetic purposes or both. *See*: DENTAL IMPLANT.

Oral implantology: *See*: IMPLANT DENTISTRY.

Oral mucosa: Epithelial lining of the oral cavity continuous with the skin of the lips and mucosa of the soft palate and pharynx, consisting of 1. Masticatory mucosa of the gingiva and hard palate, 2. Specialized mucosa of the dorsum of the tongue, and 3. Lining mucosa of the remainder of the oral cavity. *Syn*: Alveolar mucosa.

Orientation jig: *Syn*: Abutment transfer device; laboratory fabricated device for maintaining the correct position of a component transferred from the cast to the mouth.

O-ring: the doughnut-shaped, resilient overdenture attachment with the ability to bend with resistance and return to its approximate original shape; the O-ring attaches to a post with a groove or undercut area.

Oro-antral fistula: abnormal communication between the maxillary sinus and oral cavity, most often a complication after tooth extraction, but may also occur after apicectomy or due to severe periodontal disease. The teeth most frequently involved are the upper second molar, followed by the first molar. Small fistulae may close independently, but larger fistulae may require surgical closure.

Oronasal fistula: abnormal opening between the mouth and nose.

Orthodontic implant: any implant used as anchorage for tooth movement.

Orthodontics: a specialty of dentistry that deals with the study and treatment of malocclusions, tooth irregularity, disproportionate jaw relationships, or all. Also known as dentofacial orthopedics.

Osse(o): *Syn*: Osteo; pertaining to bone or containing a bony element.

Osseointegration: direct contact between living bone and a functionally loaded implant surface without interposed soft tissue at the light microscope level, with, clinically, the absence of mobility and including a sustained transfer and distribution of load from the implant to and within the bone tissue.

Osseoperception: special feeling or special sensory perception result from a changed impact force through implant-bone interface, in contrast to the cushioning effect of the skin under the socket prosthesis perhaps with intraosseous or periosteal neural endings involved.

Osseous: of the nature or quality of bone.

Osseous coagulum: mixture consisting of small bone particles and blood.

Osseous graft: *See*: BONE GRAFT.

Ossification: calcification or mineralization of bone.

Osteal: Bony, osseous.

Ostectomy: excision of bone. *See*: OSTEOPLASTY.

Osteo: *See*: OSSE(O).

Osteoblast: fully differentiated cell originating in the embryonic mesenchyme and functioning in bone tissue formation during the skeleton's early development. Osteoblasts produce inorganic salts and synthesize the collagen and glycoproteins which form the bone matrix; they develop into osteocytes.

Osteocalcin: bone-specific protein produced by the osteoblast; plays a possible role in osteoclast recruitment. Osteocalcin is an indicator of bone remodeling or mineralization.

O

Osteoclast: large, multinucleated cell arising from mononuclear precursors of the hematopoietic lineage; the osteoclast plays a role in the breakdown and resorption of osseous tissue.

Osteoconduction: bone growth by apposition from surrounding bone; during the process, an inorganic material provides scaffolding for bone growth. *See*: OSTEOINDUCTION.

Osteoconductive graft: allografts, autografts and bone substitutes that act as a conductive means for formation of osteoids, the bone matrix, especially before calcification.

Osteocyte: osteoblast embedded within the bone matrix and occupying a flat oval cavity (bone lacuna). Cells found in bone lacunae send slender cytoplasmic processes through canaliculi that make contact with processes of other osteocytes.

Osteodistraction: *See*: DISTRACTION OSTEOGENESIS.

Osteogenesis: formation and development of bone; the development of bony tissue; ossification; the histogenesis of bone.

Osteogenetic: 1. Forming bone. 2. Concerned in bone formation.

Osteogenic: *Syn*: Osteogenous; promoting the development and formation of bone exclusively from the action of osteoblasts.

Osteogenous: *See*: OSTEOGENIC.

Osteoid: 1. Resembling bone. 2. The nonmineralized bone matrix laid down by the osteoblasts and later calcified into bone with inclusion of osteoblasts as osteocytes within lacunae.

Osteoinduction: bone formation in the absence of a bony host site; new bone formation occurs as a result of osteoprogenitor cells from primitive mesenchymal cells which have come under the influence of one or more agents that emanate from the bone matrix; a process involving cellular change or cellular interaction when cells are coerced to differentiate; osteoinduction is used during autogenous bone grafting. *See*: BONE MORPHOGENETIC PROTEIN, OSTEOCONDUCTION.

Osteointegration: *See*: OSSEOINTEGRATION.

Osteomyelitis: bone inflammation from infection, which may remain localized or spread through the bone to the marrow, cortex, cancellous tissue, and periosteum.

Osteon: basic structural unit of compact bone, comprising a Haversian canal and its concentrically arranged lamellae, which may be 4 to 20, each 3μ to 7μ thick, in a single (Haversian) system, mainly directed in the long axis of the bone.

Osteonecrosis: *Syn*: Bone necrosis; the death of bone.

Osteonecrosis of the Jaw (ONJ): Literally, the death of bone in the jaws; several cases of bisphosphonate-related osteomyelitis (BON, also referred to as osteonecrosis of the jaw) have been associated with the use of the oral bisphosphonates [Fosamax (alendronate), Actonel (risedronate) and Boniva (ibandronate)] for the treatment of osteoporosis; these patients may have had other conditions that could put them at risk for developing BON.

Osteonectin: phosphoprotein in bone and blood platelets, binding both collagen and calcium and regulating mineralization.

Osteoplasty: surgical modification of bone by removal. *See*: OSTECTOMY.

Osteopontin: acidic calcium-binding phosphoprotein involved in bone mineralization with a high affinity for hydroxyapatite.

Osteoporosis: medical problem often seen in postmenopausal females and characterized by demineralization and diminution of bone mass, decreased density, and enlarged intrabony spaces.

Osteoprogenitor cell: undifferentiated cell able to transform into a bone-forming cell.

Osteopromotion: sealing off an anatomical site physically (e.g., barrier membrane) to direct bone formation and prevent soft tissue proliferation (i.e., connective tissue) from interfering with osteogenesis.

Osteoradionecrosis: bone necrosis caused by excessive exposure to radiation.

Osteotome: instrument (circular in cross-section) to expand an osteotomy apically or laterally, with or without grafting.

Osteotome lift: *See*: OSTEOTOME TECHNIQUE.

Osteotome technique: 1. Sinus grafting technique involving the careful infracturing of the maxillary sinus floor and elevation of the Schneiderian membrane via an osteotomy prepared and extended in the ridge with an osteotome. 2. The surgical expansion of an osteotomy laterally with or without grafting. *See*: RIDGE EXPANSION.

Osteotomy: 1. Site prepared in bone for the placement of an implant or graft. 2. Any surgical procedure when bone is transected or cut.

Ostium (maxillary sinus): opening connecting the maxillary sinus to the middle meatus of the nasal cavity.

Overdenture: removable partial or complete denture whose built-in secondary copings overlay (or telescope over) the primary copings, fitting over the prepared natural crowns, posts, or studs. *Syn*: Overlay denture.

Overdenture (implant): removable partial or complete denture, which may be implant-supported or implant-tissue-supported. The prosthesis is retained by attachments.

Overlay denture: *See*: OVERDENTURE.

Overload (occlusal): a reference to masticatory forces exceeding the withstanding capacity of a bone-implant interface, implant, or componentry.

Oxidized surface treatment: modification of the surface oxide properties of titanium implants by alteration of the titanium oxide layer thickness.

P

Paget disease: a malfunction in the normal process of bone growth. Normal bone growth includes a breaking down and regeneration. Paget's disease causes a malfunction in regrowth. The bone grows back weak, soft and porous, which bends easily and leads to shortening of the affected part of the body.

Palatal implant: *See*: ORTHODONTIC IMPLANT.

Palatal vault: the deepest portion of the roof of the mouth, usually found in the midline.

P

Palliative: offering relief of pain, symptoms, and stress, but not a cure.

Palpate: to examine by touching (bimanual palpation: using two hands, usually with the examined part compressed between the hands; bi-digital palpation; using two fingers, each of a different hand).

Palsy: *See*: PARALYSIS.

Panoramic radiograph: radiographic view of the maxilla and mandible extending from the left to the right glenoid fossae.

Panoramic radiography: dental tomogram that reveals the jaws, teeth, and surrounding osseous components.

Papilla: small, V-shaped gingival extensions between healthy teeth; soft tissue in the interproximal space confined by adjacent crowns in contact. *See*: INTERDENTAL PAPILLA, INTERIMPLANT PAPILLA.

Papilla-sprang incision: parasulcular incision excluding the papilla in the flap elevation.

Paracrine: of or relating to hormones or secretion released by endocrine cells into adjacent cells or surrounding tissue instead of directly into the bloodstream.

Parallel(ing) pin: *See*: DIRECTION INDICATOR.

Parallel-sided implant: *Syn*: Parallel-walled implant, Straight implant; an endosseous root-form implant with the body of the implant the same diameter at the coronal and apical ends. The platform of such an implant may have a larger diameter.

Parallel-walled implant: *See*: PARALLEL-SIDED IMPLANT.

Paralysis: *Syn*: Palsy, Paresis; loss of motor function from disease.

Paresthesia: partial loss of sensation; spontaneous or evoked abnormal sensations, not painful, often unpleasant (e.g., tingling, burning, prickling or numbness), usually caused by nerve injury and sometimes resulting from surgical procedures.

Partially edentulous: absence of one of more teeth in one portion or either the mandible or maxilla or both. To have some, but not all teeth missing.

Partial-thickness flap: a surgical flap consisting of the mucosa and submucosa but not including the periosteum. Also known as the split-thickness flap.

Particulate graft: graft consisting of particles.

Passivate: literally, to make passive; to create an oxide layer on a metal implant.

Passivation: process by which metals and alloys are made more resistant to corrosion by the creation of a thin and stable oxide layer on the external surfaces. *See*: DEPASSIVATION.

Passive: without resistance, inert.

Passive fit: fit not inducing strain between two or more implants.

Patent: open, unobstructed, not closed.

Path of placement: corridor of passivity permitting the seating or removal of a prosthesis or other intraoral device.

PDGF: *Acronym*: Platelet-derived growth factors.

Pedical flap: a skin flap that, during surgery that is elevated through connective tissue only and used to increase the width of attached gingiva.

Peer-reviewed journal: academic periodical which requires approval by panel of peers on each article submitted before publication.

Penicillin: one of the oldest and most widely used antibiotics derived from the mold, penicillium notatum, which toxic to a number of pathogens by blocking the peptidoglycan synthesis, destroying the cell wall.

Percentage bone-to-implant contact: a measure expressed as percentage of the total implant surface of the linear surface of an implant in direct contact with the bone, *See*: BONE-TO-IMPLANT CONTACT.

Perforate: to pierce or make a hole; to fenestrate.

Perforation: 1. Cortical: hole created in the cortical bone by a drill or implant. *See*: DECORTICATION. 2. Schneiderian Membrane: Tearing or creation of an opening in the maxillary sinus membrane during sinus graft surgery or following tooth extraction.

Periabutment: round the abutment.

Periapical: around or about the apex of the tooth.

Pericervical saucerization: Pathologic crestal bone loss from peri-implantitis. The bone loss is cup-shaped or saucer-like around the coronal aspect of the implant when viewed in a radiograph. *See*: PERI-IMPLANTITIS.

Peri-implant: around the implant.

Peri-implant crevicular epithelium: nonkeratinized epithelium which lines the mucosal crevice.

Peri-implant disease: inflammatory reactions in soft or hard tissues surrounding implants.

Peri-implantitis: inflammatory reactions in the hard or soft tissues, with loss of supporting bone, surrounding an implant or other implanted materials; the condition can be traumatic, ulcerative, resorptive, or exfoliative (e.g., periodontitis).

Peri-implant mucositis: reversible inflammatory reactions in the soft tissues surrounding an implant.

Periodontal biotype: two types of periodontal tissue which not only affect natural dentition, but may also affect the esthetic result in an implant-supported prosthesis. In most cases when the patient has a thick-flat periodontium, the papillae can be preserved. When the patient has the thin-scalloped periodontium, there will be papillary recession.

Periodontal dressing: a bandage and controller of hemorrhage, placed over the areas where a gingivectomy has been performed, after periodontal surgery.

Periodontal ligament: a thin, connective tissue that surrounds the root of a tooth and attaches it to the alveolar bone.

Periodontal plastic surgery: involves regenerative and reconstructive procedures designed to restore form and function in the oral cavity by eliminating gingival deficits and deformities and to also enhance esthetics. Also known as mucogingival surgery.

Periodontal pocket: abnormally deepened gum tissues surrounding a tooth that have become inflamed and infected.

Periodontal pockets make it hard to remove plaque and lead to periodontitis and bone destruction.

Periosteum: membrane of fibrous connective tissue covering all bone except at the articular surfaces (cartilaginous extremities).

Periotome: Instrument used to sever the periodontal ligament fibers prior to tooth extraction.

Permucosal: passing through or across the mucosa or epithelium.

Permucosal extension: portion of an implant extending through and beyond the epithelium. *See*: HEALING ABUTMENT.

Permucosal seal: junctional epithelium separating connective tissues from the environment outside an implant. *See*: JUNCTIONAL EPITHELIUM.

PGA: *Acronym*: Polyglycolic Acid.

Phase-1 bone regeneration: the first step toward total bone regrowth in a healing bone, involving formation of the woven bone in conjunction with a graft.

Physiologic rest position: the natural postural position of the mandible when at rest in the upright position and the condyles are in a neutral unstrained position in the mandibular fossae. Also known as postural position.

Pick-up impression: an impression made with the superstructure frame in place on the abutments in the mouth after the implant has been surgically inserted and the mouth has healed. The superstructure frame is included in the impression material, and an accurate impression of the oral mucosal tissue over the implant is obtained.

Pier abutment: *See*: INTERMEDIATE ABUTMENT.

Pilot drill: drill used to enlarge the coronal aspect of an osteotomy, so that the path of the subsequent drill can be directed.

PLA: *Acronym*: Polylactic Acid.

Placement: insertion of an implant or other device or prosthesis.

Plasma-containing growth factor: (IGF-1) the main naturally-occurring, growth factor in plasma, found in the bone matrix, that acts like insulin.

Plasma spray: implant surface treatment during which a dense or porous coating is formed after high temperature deposition of metal or ceramic powders which have been totally or partially melted and then rapidly resolidified.

Plasma spray-coated with titanium: a reliable technique for coating the surface of a titanium implant with small, irregular particles of titanium.

Plasmid: an extra-chromosomal DNA molecule capable of replicating independently of the chromosomal DNA. They occur naturally in bacteria.

Plaster: *Syn*: Dental plaster; the beta-form of calcium sulfate hemihydrate powder; it is produced by heating gypsum to eliminate water and used as modeling material in dentistry when mixed with water to reform gypsum. In guided bone regeneration, plaster can also be used as a bone graft or membrane. *See*: DENTAL STONE.

Plaster of Paris: $CaSO_4 \cdot \frac{1}{2}H_2O$ *See*: PLASTER.

P

Plastic: a description of the degree to which a material can be formed, shaped, or molded.

Plateau: an elevated flat plane or area of tissue.

Platelet: an irregular, disc-shaped, nonnucleated, disklike cytoplasmic element in the blood that assists in blood clotting. Also called blood platelet or thrombocyte. Actually fragments of large bone marrow cells called megakaryocytes.

Platelet-derived growth factors (PDGF): growth factors released by platelets which initiate connective tissue healing (e.g., bone regeneration and repair). These factors also increase mitogenesis, angiogenesis, and macrophage activation.

Platelet gel: referring to an Autogenous Hematopoetic Tissue Graft a Surgeon creates from harvesting your own natural healing factors (stem cells, growth factors, platelets and white cells) from your blood.

Platelet-poor plasma (PPP): lesser concentration of active platelets that remain after the separation process to derive platelet-rich plasma.

Platelet-rich plasma (PRP): autologous product derived from whole blood through the process of gradient density centrifugation, the purpose of which is derive a substance able to incorporate high concentrations of growth factors PDGF, TGF- El, TGF-L2, IGF, VEGF, FGF-1, and fibrin into a graft mixture.

Platform: *Syn*: Prosthetic table, Restorative platform, Seating surface; the coronal aspect of an implant to which abutments, components, and prostheses may be connected.

Platform switching: *Syn*: Abutment swapping; using an abutment with a diameter narrower than that of the implant platform and, so, moving the implant-abutment junction away from the edge of the platform.

Pneumatization: a process by which air-filled cavities become an increasing part of a body. *See*: PNEUMATIZED MAXILLARY SINUS.

Pneumatized maxillary sinus: maxillary sinus enlargement; gradual thinning of the sinus walls as a result of the increase in size of the maxillary sinus, usually the result of aging and loss of maxillary teeth (and masticatory forces).

Polish: to treat with abrasives of graduated fineness (machined finish).

Polished surface: machined (smoother) surface.

Polishing cap: component connected to the abutment's apical part to protect the base and allow the lab to polish the prosthesis and abutment without excessive reduction of the base diameter or rounding of edges.

Polyglactin: multifilament braided purified lactides and glycolides used as absorbable sutures or membranes.

Polyglycolic Acid (PGA): polymer of glycolic acid used for absorbable sutures or membranes.

Polylactic Acid (PLA): polymer of lactic acid used for absorbable sutures or membranes.

Polymer: natural or synthetic substance composed of giant molecules formed from smaller molecules of the same substance.

Polymorphonuclear leukocyte: a type of white blood cell with a nucleus that is divided so that the cell looks to have multiple nuclei.

Polysulfide rubber: an elastomeric impression material; Thiokol.

Polytetrafluoroethylene: a synthetic fluoropolymer commonly known as Teflon. Used in a variety of surgical material such as guided tissue regeneration.

Polyvinylsiloxane: elastomeric impression material.

Pontic: a false tooth in a dental bridge.

Porosity: having minute openings or pores.

Porous: characterized by pores or voids within a structure (e.g., grafting material, implant surface).

Porous coralline hydroxyapatite: a bone substitute from Porite coral shown to facilitate growth of bone into the desired shape, that is nonresorbable but osteoconductive.

Porous surface: *See*: PLASMA SPRAYED, SINTERED (POROUS) SURFACE.

Posterior palatal seal, postdam: postpalatal seal; the seal at the posterior border of a denture.

Posterior superior alveolar artery: one of three arteries (along with infraorbital and posterior lateral nasal arteries) supplying the maxillary sinus, all of which are ultimate branches of the maxillary artery. During lateral approach sinus elevation surgery, any of these arteries may be encountered.

Postpalatal seal: *See*: POSTERIOR PALATAL SEAL.

PPP: *Acronym*: Platelet-poor plasma.

Prefabricated abutment: machine-manufactured abutment.

Prefabricated coping: thimble prepared to fit an abutment.

Prefabricated cylinder: component made of a noble alloy and connecting to an implant or abutment; to form a custom abutment for a cement-retained or screw-retained prosthesis, a compatible alloy is cast to the cylinder.

Preload: energy transferred to a screw after torque is applied during tightening. The result of such stretching is that the screw threads are tightly secured to the screw's mating counterpart, holding them together by producing a clamping force between the screw head and seat.

Prepable abutment: abutment prepared and modified from its original manufactured design.

Preprosthetic surgery: surgery performed to improve the prognosis of planned prostheses.

Press-fit: retention of a root-form implant from close proximity of the bone; alternatively, a reference to the retention of certain components into the implant. *See*: FRICTION-FIT.

Primary bone: *See*: BONE.

Primary closure: bringing the flaps of a wound together to prevent tension and to enable atraumatic suturing. *See*: HEALING BY FIRST (PRIMARY) INTENTION.

Primary implant failure: *See*: EARLY IMPLANT FAILURE.

Primary stability: *See*: INITIAL STABILITY.

Primitive bone: *See*: BONE.

Prions: proteinaceous infectious particles which show marked resistance to conventional inactivation procedures, including

P

irradiation, boiling, dry heat, and chemical treatment; these particles cause and transmit bovine spongiform encephalopathy and similar encephalopathies. However, other deactivating agents can be successfully used against prions, including denaturing organic solvents, chaotropic agents, and alkali.

Probing depth: as measured by a periodontal probe, the distance from the free mucosal or gingival margin to the base of the pen-implant or periodontal sulcus.

Probing depths: pocket depths adjacent to implants or teeth.

Profiler (bone): burs (with different profiler diameters to accommodate a desired component diameter) for removing bone around the platform of a root-form implant, thus allowing the connection of components to the implant.

Profilometer: device used to trace and record the roughness of a surface at high magnification.

Progenitor cell: undifferentiated cell able to transform into one or more types of cells.

Prognathism: a protruding mandible.

Prognosis: a prediction of the outcome of therapy.

Progressive loading: placing a series of increasingly hard prostheses into function, usually beginning with acrylic and ending with porcelain; gradually increasing the application of load on a prosthesis and implant.

Proprioception: ability of sensory nerves to determine the position of body parts.

Prospective study: study planned to observe events that have not yet occurred.

Prosthesis: *Syn*: Restoration; artificial replacement of a missing part of the body; artificial device used to substitute for a lost or underfunctioning body part.

Prosthetic: artificial.

Prosthetic screw: *Syn*: Retaining screw; screw used in a prosthetic reconstruction to connect a prosthesis to an implant or an abutment.

Prosthetic table: *See*: PLATFORM.

Prosthodontic abutment: *See*: ABUTMENT.

Prosthodontics: art and science of diagnosis, treatment, maintenance, and follow-up care of patients requiring artificial dentures or oromaxillofacial parts.

Protocol: details for a proposed activity, such as surgical protocol, prosthetic protocol, and research protocol.

Provisional implant: *See*: TRANSITIONAL IMPLANT.

Provisionalization: the process of creating a temporary and alterable prosthesis.

Provisional prosthesis/restoration: *See*: INTERIM PROSTHESIS/ RESTORATION.

Provisional restoration: prostheses made for temporary purposes.

Proximal: toward the center of a body.

PRP: *Acronym*: Platelet-rich plasma.

Pterygoid implant: root-form implant originating near the former second maxillary molar; its end point encroaches in the scaphoid fossa of the sphenoid bone. The implant follows an intrasinusal trajectory in a dorsal and mesio-cranial direction, perforating the posterior sinus wall and the pterygoid plates.

Pterygoid notch: groove at the pyramidal process of the palatine bone between the pterygoid plates and the maxillary tuberosity.

Pterygomaxillary notch: bony groove between the maxillary tuberosity and the pterygoid bone (lesser sphenoidal wing).

Punch technique: exposure of the implant by the removal of a circular piece of soft tissue over a submerged implant; the incision is approximately the diameter of the implant platform.

P-value: probability that a test statistic will assume a value as extreme as or more extreme than that seen under the assumption that the null hypothesis is true.

Quadrant: any one of four parts created by dividing an object with two right-angled intersecting lines.

R

RAD: radiation absorbed dose.

Radicular: referring to root.

Radiograph: an X-ray.

Radiographic guide: *See*: RADIOGRAPHIC TEMPLATE.

Radiographic marker: radiopaque structure of known dimension, or a material incorporated in or applied to a radiographic template to yield positional or dimensional information.

Radiographic template: guide used for diagnosis and planning phases for dental implants; the template is derived from a diagnostic wax-up and worn during the radiographic exposure to show the tooth position to nearby anatomical structures.

Radiolucent: the quality of appearing dense or black on exposed X-ray film; allowing the passage of X rays or other radiation.

Radiopaque: the quality of appearing light or white on exposed X-ray film; capable of blocking X-rays.

Ramus endosteal implant: blade implant designed for placement in the anterior ramus of the mandible.

Ramus frame endosteal implant: three-component blade complex composed of an anterior foot and bilateral ramus extensions.

Ramus frame implant: full-arch mandibular implant with a tripodal design consisting of a horizontal supragingival connecting bar with endosseous units placed into the two rami and symphyseal area.

Ramus graft: bone graft harvested from the lateral aspect of the ascending ramus of the mandible, consisting of mostly cortical bone.

R

Radionecrosis: osteonecrosis due to excessive exposure to radiation. Typically seen to occur in patients who have undergone chemotherapy for tumors that were located anywhere from the neck up.

Radiopaque marker: a marker used to interpret an object's length, angulation or localization within an x-ray image. It is made of metal or any other radiopaque material, meaning that does not let x-rays or other types of radiation penetrate.

Ramus: the posterior vertical part of the mandible on each side which extends from the corpus to the condyle, and makes a joint at the temple.

Random controlled trial: prospective study detailing the effects of a particular procedure or material; in such a study, subjects are randomly assigned to either test or control groups. The former receives the procedure or material while the latter receives a standard procedure, or material, a different test procedure, or a placebo.

RAP: *Acronym*: Regional acceleratory phenomenon.

Ratchet: wrench for threaded implants to facilitate final implant seating.

RBM: *Acronym*: Resorbable blast media.

Reactive bone: *See*: BONE.

Reamer: Tool for finishing the mating surface of a metal cylinder/coping, specifically the screw seat interface.

Receptor sites: areas in the maxillary mucosa into which are nestled the heads of intramucosal inserts.

Recipient site: *See*: HOST SITE; site which receives a soft or hard tissue graft.

Recombinant human bone morphogenetic protein (rhBMP): osteoinductive protein produced by recombinant DNA technology.

Record base: a temporary form representing the base of a denture and used to help establish maxillomandibular relation records for facilitating trial placement in the oral cavity. Also known as baseplate.

Re-entry: surgical reopening of a site to improve or observe results from the initial procedure.

Reflection: elevation or folding back of the mucoperiosteum to expose the underlying bone.

Refractory: resistant to treatment.

Regenerate: *Syn*: Distraction zone; tissue forming between gradually separated bone segments in distraction osteogenesis.

Regenerate maturation: completion of mineralization and remodeling of the regenerate tissue.

Regeneration: reproduction or reconstitution of a lost or injured part to its original state; restoration of body parts after trauma. *See*: REPAIR.

Regional acceleratory phenomenon (RAP): local response to a stimulus in which tissues form two to 10 times more rapidly than the normal regeneration process. The duration and intensity are directly proportional to the kind and amount of stimulus as well as to the site where it was produced.

Reimplantation: act of reinserting a tooth into the alveolar socket from which it has been removed.

Rejection: immunological response of incompatibility in a transplanted organ or implanted device.

Releasing incision: an incision made to allow for periodontal flap repositioning and/or mobility for suture closure.

Remodel: morphologic change in bone as it adapts to environmental stimuli.

Remodeling (bone): turnover of bone in small packets by basic multicellular units (BMUs) of bone remodeling.

Removable prosthesis: restoration that the patient can remove partially (RPD: Removable partial denture) or completely (RCD: Removable complete denture). *See*: DENTURE, FIXED PROSTHESIS.

Removal torque: rotational force applied to remove the implant from its placement within the bone.

Removal torque value (RTV): *Syn*: Reverse torque value; measure of rotational force to rupture the bone-implant interface of a root-form implant.

Repair: healing of a wound by tissue that does not fully restore the architecture or function of the lost part. *See*: REGENERATION.

Replica: *See*: ANALOG.

Replicate: to reproduce.

Residual ridge: remnant of the alveolar process and soft tissue covering after teeth removal.

Resilient: springing back into shape or position.

Resin: a compound made by condensation or polymerization of low-molecular-weight organic compounds, clear to translucent yellow or brown, which begins in a highly viscous state and hardens with treatment. Typically, resin is soluble in alcohol, but not in water.

Resonance frequency analysis (RFA): technique for clinical measurement of implant stability/mobility, registering by means of a transducer attached to the abutment or implant, which records the resonance frequency arising from the implant-bone interface (change in amplitude over induced frequency band).

Resorbable: ability of an autogenous graft to dissolve physiologically. *See*: BIOABSORBABLE.

Resorbable blast media (RBM): surface treatment obtained by blasting the implant surface with a biocompatible material (e.g., tricalcium phosphate).

Resorpable membrane: a natural or synthetic absorbable membrane that goes over the bone grafting before dental implantation, that does not need to have a second surgery to remove it.

Resorption: loss of substance or bone by physiologic (natural) or pathologic means. *See*: BONE RESORPTION.

Restoration: *See*: PROSTHESIS.

Restorative platform: *See*: PLATFORM.

Retainer: any type of clasp, attachment, or device used for the fixation or stabilization of a prosthesis.

Retaining screw: *See*: PROSTHETIC SCREW.

Rethreading: repair of the damaged internal threads of a root-form implant using a tap instrument.

Retractor: all the instruments used to keep a patient's mouth open wide and steady during procedures.

Retrievability: a reference to the likelihood of removing a prosthesis undamaged.

Retromolar pad: mass of tissue (frequently pear-shaped) located at the distal termination of the mandibular residual ridge and composed of the retromolar papilla and the retromolar glandular prominence.

Retrospective study: study designed to observe events that have already occurred.

Retrusion: a posterior position.

Reverse articulation: full arch crossbite; class III malocclusion.

Reverse torque test (RTT): an assessment of the extent of osseointegration, specifically the shear strength at the bone-implant interface; the test include the applying of rotational force in a direction opposite to that used to place the implant.

Reverse torque value: *See*: REMOVAL TORQUE VALUE.

Revolutions per minute (rpm): unit of rotational speed at which a bur or drill turns.

RFA: *Acronym*: Resonance frequency analysis.

rhBMP: *Acronym*: Recombinant human bone morphogenetic protein.

Ridge: remainder of the alveolar process after teeth extraction. *See*: ALVEOLAR PROCESS, RESIDUAL RIDGE.

Ridge, alveolar: alveolar process and its soft-tissue covering that remain after teeth are removed.

Ridge atrophy: decrease in volume of the ridge caused by bone resorption.

Ridge augmentation: increasing the dimension of the existing alveolar ridge morphology.

Ridge crest: highest continuous surface of the alveolar ridge.

Ridge defect: deficiency in the contour of the edentulous ridge, both vertical (apicocoronal) and/or horizontal (buccolingual, mesiodistal) direction.

Ridge expansion: surgical widening of the residual ridge with osteotomes and/or chisels in the lateral direction (buccolingually), in order to accommodate the insertion of an implant and/or bone graft.

Ridge lap: portion of a pontic which opposes the edentulous crest (sanitary ridge lap; bullet-shaped ridge lap).

Ridge mapping: creating a diagnostic cast by transposing information obtained after penetrating anesthetized soft tissue with a graduated probe or caliper at several sites; shape of the residual ridge is reproduced by trimming back the stone of the cast to the corresponding depth of soft tissue. *See*: RIDGE SOUNDING.

Ridge preservation: *Syn*: Extraction socket graft, Socket graft, Socket preservation; immediate placement of a grafting material or any procedure (e.g., Guided Bone Regeneration) performed on the extraction socket following tooth extraction in order to conserve the bone and soft tissue contours by avoiding bone resorption with a resultant ridge defect.

Ridge resorption: the loss of bone in an edentulous area. *See*: RESIDUAL RIDGE.

Ridge sounding: *Syn*: Bone sounding, Sounding; penetration of anesthetized soft tissue to determine the topography of the underlying bone. *See*: RIDGE MAPPING.

Ridge splitting: *See*: RIDGE EXPANSION.

Rigid fixation: absence of observed mobility.

Risk factor: condition shown to negatively affect the success of a treatment modality.

Residual ridge resorption: the resorption of alveolar bone after tooth removal.

Root form: similar in shape to a dental root.

Root form endosteal dental implant: endosseous implant, circular in cross-section, and root-shaped; it is supported from a vertical expanse of bone; implants can be in the form of spirals, cones, rhomboids, and cylinders. Additionally, such implants can be smooth, fluted, finned, threaded, perforated, solid, hollow, or vented. Finally, these implants can be coated or textured; they are generally available in submergible and non- submergible forms in a variety of biocompatible materials.

Root-form implant: *See*: ROOT FORM ENDOSTEAL DENTAL IMPLANT.

Root-form implants shear loading: forces delivered in the plane of the long axis of an implant.

Rotation: the action of turning on an axis.

Rough surface: *See*: TEXTURED SURFACE.

Round bur: circular bur for marking site for an osteotomy or to decorticate bone. It may also be used in the outline of a lateral window access for sinus grafting.

Rpm: *Acronym*: Revolutions per minute.

Rugae: ridges and folds running horizontally in the anterior palatal mucosa.

R-value: two-dimensional roughness parameter calculated from the experimental profiles after filtering. Ra: arithmetic average of the absolute value of all points of the profile, also called central line average height. Rt: maximum peak-to-valley height of the entire measurement trace.

S

Saddle: part of a complete or partial denture to which the teeth are attached and which rests on the ridge.

Sagittal plane: any vertical section parallel to the median plane of the body, dividing it into right and left parts.

Sandblasting: grit blasting of an implant surface with sand.

Saucerization: *See*: PERICERVICAL SAUCERIZATION.

Saucerization: pericervical implant bone loss adjacent to all implants.

Scaffold: framework or armature; three-dimensional biocompatible construct (may be seeded with cells) acting as a framework and providing a structure on which tissue grows. It may be replaced by natural tissue.

Scalloped implant: a root-form implant with the level of the implant-abutment junction more coronal interproximally than facially or lingually.

Scanning microscopy: an image recorded point-by-point by means of a beam of electrons and projected to a television monitor.

Scanographic template: radiographic template used for CT-scanning. *See*: RADIOGRAPHIC TEMPLATE.

Scar: fibrous tissue which replaces normal tissues after healing.

Schneiderian membrane: *Syn*: Sinus membrane (maxillary); layer of pseudostratified ciliated columnar epithelium cells lining the maxillary sinus. *See*: PERFORATION.

Screw endosteal dental implant: Threaded root-form implant, parallel-sided or tapered. *See*: ROOT-FORM IMPLANT, THREADED IMPLANT, ENDOSTEAL ROOT FORM IMPLANT.

Screw implant: *See*: ROOT-FORM IMPLANT.

Screw joint: junction of two parts held together by a screw (e.g., implant-abutment screw joint).

Screw loosening: prosthetic complication occurring when a screw loses its preload, causing the restoration or abutment to loosen.

Screw-retained: description of an abutment or a prosthesis whose retention is accomplished by a screw. *See*: CEMENT-RETAINED.

Screw tap: *See*: TAP.

SD: *Acronym*: Standard deviation.

Sealing screw: *See*: HYGIENE CAP.

Seating surface: *See*: PLATFORM.

Secondary closure: *See*: HEALING BY SECOND (SECONDARY) INTENTION.

Secondary Implant failure: *See*: LATE IMPLANT FAILURE.

Second-stage implant surgery: subperiosteal implant: reopening of the tissue and placement of the infrastructure that was constructed after the first-stage surgery; endosteal submerged implants: re-exposure of the portion of the implant that receives the attachment or abutment.

Second-stage permucosal abutment: *See*: HEALING ABUTMENT.

Second-stage surgery: *See*: STAGE-TWO SURGERY.

Self-tapping: feature of the apical aspect of a threaded implant or screw to create its thread path in the bone.

Semiadjustable articulator: adjustable device simulating jaw movements so that it conforms to actual mandibular functions.

Semiprecious metal alloy: mixture of base metal(s) with gold, platinum, or both.

Senile atrophy: a condition of tissue or organ losing morphology or function because of the age of the patient.

Septum: a compartment or wall between two cavities.

Septum (maxillary sinus): *Syn*: Underwood cleft; spine-like bony structure or web formation in some maxillary sinuses which may divide the inferior portion of the sinus into sections. *See*: ALVEOLAR RECESS.

Sequestration: to separate a portion of necrotic from the whole surrounding bone.

Serum CTX: a marker of bone resorption (serum C-terminal cross-linking telopeptide of type I collagen); serum CTX testing may be used to help determine the stage of Biosphosphonate-Induced Osteonecrosis of the jaws.

Set screw: prosthetic or retention screw, lab-prepared in the prescribed location on the prosthesis (usually lingual); the set screw joins the crown to the abutment or the superstructure to the mesostructure and may also complement a cement-retained restoration.

Sharpey connective tissue fibers: periosteal connective tissue collagen becomes incorporated into the matrix that is being laid down by the surface osteoblasts and serves to anchor the periosteum to the cementum.

Shear stress: stress caused by a load that tends to slide one portion of object over another. The forces applied in such stress are toward one another but not in the same straight line. *See*: STRESS, ROOT-FORM IMPLANTS SHEAR LOADING.

Shoulder finish line: the casting endpoint on a tooth after its preparation.

Simultaneous placement: insertion of a root- form implant in conjunction with another surgical procedure performed at the same site (e.g., grafting).

Single crystal sapphire: material for implantation composed of a single crystalline alpha aluminum oxide identical in crystalline structure to a gem sapphire.

Single-stage implant: *See*: ONE-STAGE IMPLANT.

Single-stage surgery: single stage (implant) surgery is to graft or insert into the body in one single step.

Sinter: to fuse together; in biomaterials, with hydraulic pressure.

Sintered: treated by sintering. *See*: SINTERING.

Sintered (porous) surface: implant surface produced when spherical powders of metallic or ceramic materials become a coherent mass with the metallic core of the implant body; porous surfaces are characterized by pore size, pore shape, pore volume, and pore depth, which are affected by the size of the spherical particles and the temperature and pressure conditions of the sintering chamber.

Sintering: heating a powder below the melting point of any component to permit agglomeration and welding of particles by diffusion alone, with or without applied pressure.

Sinus: air space within bone.

Sinus augmentation: the use of open or osteotome techniques for placement of bone grafting materials in the antral floor. *See*: SINUS GRAFT.

Sinus elevation: *See*: SINUS GRAFT.

Sinus floor elevation: antroplasty; sinus floor augmentation; bone grafting via a modified Caldwell-Luc approach to improve the posterior maxilla for placement of an endosteal implant; often preferable to subantral augmentation.

Sinus graft: *Syn*: Maxillary antroplasty, Sinus augmentation, Sinus elevation, Sinus lift, Subantral augmentation; augmentation of the antral floor with autogenous bone and/or bone to improve conditions for placement of a dental implant.

Sinus perforation: when a direct connection between the sinus and mouth is created by a perforation of the maxillary sinus membrane following a tooth extraction or a sinus grafting procedure.

Sinusitis (maxillary): inflammation of the sinus; signs include sensitivity of teeth to percussion, fever, and facial swelling. Symptoms: nasal congestion, postnasal discharge, facial pain/headache, rhinorrhea, halitosis, popping of ears, and muffled hearing.

Sinus lift: *See*: SINUS GRAFT.

Sinus membrane (maxillary): *See*: SCHNEIDERIAN MEMBRANE.

Sinus pneumatization (maxillary): maxillary sinus enlargement; gradual thinning of the sinus walls as a result of the increase in size of the maxillary sinus, usually the result of aging and loss of maxillary teeth (and masticatory forces).

Site development: augmenting the quantity and quality of soft and/or hard tissues prior to implant placement.

Sleeper implant: an implant that is nonfunctioning, nonprotruding through the mucoperiosteum into the oral cavity that serves in to fix a fracture or to conserve a bone.

Sluiceway: a slot or passage permitting the passage of fluids.

Smile line: the gingival line that follows the contour of the lower lip imaginary when the patient is smiling.

Socket: an alveolus; depression such as those placed in special wrenches.

Socket graft: *See*: RIDGE PRESERVATION.

Socket preservation: *See*: RIDGE.

Soft tissue cast: cast with the implant laboratory analog platform surrounded by an elastic mucosal simulating material.

Solid: dense mass.

Solid screw: root-form threaded implant of circular cross-section with no vents or holes penetrating the body.

Sounding: *See*: RIDGE SOUNDING.

Spark erosion: *See*: ELECTRIC DISCHARGE METHOD.

Specialized mucosa: *See*: ORAL MUCOSA.

Sphincter: round band of muscle designed to permit the closing of a passageway.

Spirochete: a microscopic bacterial organism of the order Spirochaetales, many of which are pathogenic, causing syphilis, relapsing fever, yaws, and periodontitis.

Splint *(noun):* device designed to hold or stabilize weakened or injured hard tissues; a series of connected crowns.

Splint *(verb):* to apply a supporting device to aid weakened or injured hard tissues.

Splinting: joining of two or more abutments into a unit; joining two or more teeth or implants into a rigid or nonrigid unit via fixed or removable restorations or devices.

Split crest technique: *See*: RIDGE EXPANSION.

Split ridge technique: *See*: RIDGE EXPANSION.

Split thickness graft: slice of epithelium taken for transplantation.

Spongy bone: *See*: BONE.

Staged protocol: treatment sequence involving the completion of one procedure followed by another at a later date.

Stage-one surgery: *Syn*: First-stage dental implant surgery; surgical procedure consisting of placing an endosseous implant in the bone and suturing the soft tissue over the implant to submerge the implant for healing.

Stage-two surgery: *Syn*: Second-stage surgery; surgical procedure consisting of exposing a submerged implant to the oral environment by connecting an abutment extruding through the soft tissue.

Standard abutment: machined titanium, cylindrical abutment to support a screw-retained prosthesis. *See*: HYBRID PROSTHESIS.

Standard deviation (SD): statistical term indicating the variability or dispersion of a distribution of scores, the more scores clustering around the mean, the smaller the standard deviation.

Staple implant: implant inserted via a submental skin incision through the inferior border of the mandible and exiting through the alveolar ridge as one or multiple abutments. The implant's retention is established by a screw fastened foot plate. *See*: MANDIBULAR STAPLE IMPLANT.

Static: body at rest.

Stem cells: cells potentially developing into a significant series ending with red blood cells.

Stem cell: undifferentiated cell of embryogenic or adult origin that can undergo unlimited division and give rise to one or several different cell types.

Stent: a prosthetic device used to influence and guide the healing of soft tissues; surgical device used to keep a graft in place or protect a surgical site during initial healing; incorrect term for guide, splint, or template. *Syn*: Radiographic template, Surgical guide.

Stepping implant: endosseous, root-form implant with parallel walls of different diameter joined to form a step.

Stereolithographic guide: guide generated from a CAM according to a software planned implant placement.

Stereolithography: *Syn*: Three-dimensional imaging, Three-dimensional modeling; method for creating a three-dimensional model using lasers driven by CAD software from CT-scan information. The model is used for surgical planning and the generation of a guide.

Sterile technique: surgical procedure performed under sterile conditions, under operating room conditions and following operating room protocol for setup, instrument transfer and handling, and personnel movement. Clinicians wear surgical scrubs, head covers, shoe covers, and sterile gowns; a standard technique in which an aseptic area is established and maintained to a specific conclusion (e.g., the proper sterilization of instruments, drapes, gowns, gloves, and surgical area); the systematic maintenance of asepsis throughout an implant insertion procedure. *See*: CLEAN TECHNIQUE.

Sterilization: complete elimination of microbial life; caution must be used during sterilization to preserve the integrity and properties of the implant.

Stomatognathic: relating to the jaws and mouth.

Straight abutment: *See*: NONANGULATED ABUTMENT.

Straight/angled abutments: *See*: ABUTMENT.

Straight implant: *See*: PARALLEL-SIDED IMPLANT.

Strain: an object's dimensional change after being subjected to stress; change in an object's length after application of stress.

Stress: mechanical tensile force: the form divided by perpendicular cross-sectional area over which force is applied; force or load applied to an object. Types of stress include: bending, compressive, shear, tensile, and torsion. *See*: BENDING STRESS, COMPRESSIVE STRESS, SHEAR STRESS, TENSILE STRESS, TORSION STRESS.

Stress breaker: device designed to ameliorate abutment stresses via soft, compliant materials, springs, or hinges.

Stress broken: a description of the after effects of having used devices to relieve the abutment teeth of all or part of the occlusal forces.

Stress concentration: point where stress is substantially higher because of the geometry of the stressed object or the point of force application.

Stripped threads: a description of jammed threads of a screw or the internal threads of a root-form implant which have been bent, broken, or otherwise damaged.

Stripping: a reference to damage (i.e., distortion or obliteration) done to the internal threads of an implant or abutment.

Subantral augmentation: *See*: SINUS GRAFT.

Subcrestal implant placement: *See*: CRESTAL IMPLANT PLACEMENT.

Sublingual artery: an artery with origin in the anterior margin of the hyglossus and runs from the forward between the genioglossus and mylohyoideus to the sublingual gland.

Submerged implant: implant covered by soft tissue and (so) isolated from the oral cavity.

Submergible: able to be buried.

Submergible implant: *See*: TWO-STAGE IMPLANT.

Submersible endosteal implant: *See*: ENDOSTEAL (ENDOSSEOUS) IMPLANT.

Submersible implant: buried or partially buried implant.

Submucosal inserts: *See*: INTRAMUCOSAL INSERT.

Submucous cleft palate: bony cleft not readily detected by clinical examination.

Subnasal elevation: a surgical technique to enhance anterior bone height in the anterior maxilla.

Subperiosteal dental implant: framework specifically constructed (complete-arch, unilateral, or universal) to fit supporting areas of the mandible or maxillae with permucosal extensions for a prosthesis; the framework consists of permucosal extensions with or without connecting bars and struts (peripheral, primary, and secondary).

Subperiosteal dental implant abutment: *See*: ABUTMENT.

Subperiosteal dental implant substructure: *See*: INFRASTRUCTURE.

Subperiosteal dental implant superstructure: *See*: OVERDENTURE.

Subperiosteal implant: implant consisting of a customized casting, made of a surgical grade metal, which rests on the surface of bone and under the periosteum. Prosthetic retention is accomplished by permucosal abutments, posts, and intraoral bars. 1. Complete: for a completely edentulous arch 2. Unilateral: located on one side of the posterior mandible or maxilla. 3. Circumferential: bypasses remaining teeth or implants.

Subtracted surface: *Syn*: Subtractive surface treatment; alteration of an implant surface by material removal. *See*: ADDED SURFACE, TEXTURED SURFACE.

Subtraction radiography: technique for detecting radiographic density change at two points in time to determine bone formation or loss.

Subtractive surface treatment: *See*: SUBTRACTED SURFACE.

Success criteria: conditions established by a study protocol for evaluating a procedure's effectiveness.

Success rate: percentage of success of a procedure or device (e.g., implant) in a study or clinical trial based on success criteria as defined by the study protocol. *See*: SURVIVAL RATE.

Sulcular epithelium: *Syn*: Crevicular epithelium; nonkeratinized epithelium of the mucosal sulcus surrounding implants and teeth.

Superstructure: prosthesis that attaches to an implant's abutments or an intermediary casting, called a mesostructure; prosthesis supported by implants with or without a mesostructure.

Suppuration: pus formation.

Supracrestal implant placement: *See*: CRESTAL IMPLANT PLACEMENT.

Surface alteration: modification of an implant surface by treatment. *See*: ADDED SURFACE, SUBTRACTED SURFACE.

Surface characteristics (implant): implant topography, defined by form (the largest structure or profile), waviness, and roughness (the smallest irregularities in the surface). Waviness and roughness are often referred to collectively as texture. Implant surfaces are usually designated as machined or textured. *See*: MACHINED SURFACE, TEXTURED SURFACE.

Surface roughness: qualitative and quantitative features of an implant surface determined two- dimensionally by contact stylus profilometry (*See*: R VALUE) or three-dimensionally by confocal laser scanner (*See*: S VALUE). *See*: SURFACE.

Surgical bed: site prepared to receive a graft.

Surgical guide: guide derived from the diagnostic wax-up to assist in the preparation for placement and the placement of implants; the surgical guide determines drilling position and angulation; template fabricated to reveal implant osteotomies to the surgeon.

Surgical indexing: record for registering the position of an implant at stage-one or stage-two surgery.

Surgical jaw relationship, subperiosteal: registration of the vertical dimension in centric relationship of the exposed superior surface of the mandibular or maxillary bone with the opposing arch, providing intermaxillary registration for determination of abutment height of a subperiosteal implant framework.

Surgical navigation: real time computer technology used to aid in the intraoperative navigation of surgical instruments and operation site, allowing for precise operation site localization before and during surgery.

Surgical occlusal rim, subperiosteal: conventional occlusion rim with a base adapted for accurate recording of the surgical vertical-centric relations.

Surgical template: *See*: SURGICAL GUIDE.

Survival rate: percentage of implant success in a study or clinical trial; success is most often defined as implants functioning according to predetermined criteria. *See*: SUCCESS RATE.

Suture: *verb*: to joining together by sewing.

Suturing: wound closure with thread.

S value: three-dimensional roughness parameter calculated from topographical images. Sa: arithmetic average of the absolute value of all points of the profile, a height descriptive parameter. Scx: space descriptive parameter. Sdr: developed surface area ratio.

Swage: to press or hammer malleable material to adapt it to an underlying model or form.

Symphysis: immovable dense midline articulation of the right and left halves of the adult mandible.

Syngeneic graft: *See*: ISOGRAFT.

System (implant): 1. product line of implants (often representing a specific concept, inventor, or patent) with specific surgical protocol and matching prosthetic components. *See*: CONFIGURATION. 2. ISO definition: "Dental implant components that are designed to mate together. It consists of the necessary parts and instruments to complete the implant body placement and abutment components." (ISO 10451).

T

Tack: *Syn*: Fixation tack. Metal or bioabsorbable pin with a flat head to secure the barrier membrane position during guided bone regeneration.

Tap: *Syn*: Threader, Threadformer. 1. Bone tap: Device to create a threaded channel in bone for a fixation screw or prior to the insertion of an implant. 2. Metal tap: instrument (harder than titanium) used for rethreading the damaged internal threads of an implant.

Tapered implant: endosseous, root-form implant (threaded or nonthreaded) with a wider diameter coronally than apically; the sides converge apically.

Tapping: creating a threaded channel in bone with a bone tap for placing a fixation screw or prior to the insertion of an implant (also known as pretapping).

TCP: *Acronym*: Tricalcium phosphate.

Team approach: Use a multi-disciplinary team approach that combines the collaboration of various healthcare providers in the post-operative management of a patient with dental implants.

Teeth in an Hour: Nobel Biocare trademark which reflects the general advancements in technology (e.g., CT scans, CAD/CAM software) and procedure (e.g., timely prosthesis fabrication, computer-guided surgery via templates) for using dental implants to provide edentulous patients (upper, lower, or complete) with functionally esthetic tooth function in minimal time. The technique employs pre-made (temporary or final) prosthetics ready for use at the time of surgery, eliminating multiple surgeries and visits.

Telescopic coping: thin metal covering or cap fitted over the prepared tooth or implant abutment to accept a secondary or overlay crown or prosthesis.

Telescopic denture: denture fitting over retentive extensions (tooth or implant borne). See: OVERDENTURE.

Template: guide. *See*: RADIOGRAPHIC TEMPLATE, STEREOLITHOGRAPHIC GUIDE, SURGICAL GUIDE.

Temporary abutment: *Syn*: Temporary cylinder; abutment for the fabrication of an interim restoration, which may be cemented on the temporary abutment. The temporary abutment may be incorporated in the interim restoration as screw-retained.

Temporary cylinder: *See*: TEMPORARY ABUTMENT.

Temporary healing cuff: *See*: HEALING ABUTMENT.

Temporary prosthesis/restoration: *See*: INTERIM PROSTHESIS/RESTORATION.

Tensile stress: stress caused by a load (two forces applied away from one another in the same straight line) tending to stretch or elongate an object; pulling force. *See*: STRESS.

Tension: pulling or drawing away.

Tension-free wound closure: closure for a post-operative wound that can be done by without flap tension.

Tenting screw: metal screw used to support a barrier membrane to maintain a space under the membrane for guiding bone regeneration.

Tent pole procedure: a surgical procedure whereby the periosteum and soft tissue matrix are elevated through the use of dental implants, creating a tenting effect, which prevent graft resorption. Tent pole procedure also offers predictable long-term reconstruction of the severely resorbed mandible without complications.

Tetracycline: antibiotic used to treat bacterial infections, typically used to treat rhinogenic infections.

Textured surface: machined implant surface that has been altered or modified by addition or reduction. *See*: ADDED SURFACE, MACHINED SURFACE, SUBTRACTED SURFACE, SURFACE CHARACTERISTICS (IMPLANT).

Texturing: process by which the surface area of an implant is increased. *See*: TEXTURED SURFACE.

TGF-b: abbreviation for the Transforming Growth Factor Beta, one of two classes of transforming growth factors which are found in hematopoietic tissue and stimulate bone healing and regeneration.

Thick flat periodontium: Also know as the periodontal biotype, this thick, flat, short and wide tooth and its supporting structure, including the cementum, the periodontal membrane, the bone of the alveolar process, and the gums.

Thermal expansion: enlargement of a material by heat.

Thermoplastic: heat labile.

Thin scalloped periodontium: a thin, filed-down ends of a tooth, the supporting structures of the teeth including the cementum, the periodontal membrane, the bone of the alveolar process, and the gums.

Thread: extruding feature of the body of certain implants. Geometric characteristics include thread depth, thickness, pitch, face angle, and helix angle. Basic thread geometries include: V-thread, buttress thread, and power (square) thread.

Threaded implant: endosseous, root-form implant with threads similar to a screw, also known as a screw-shaped implant; sides may be parallel-sided or tapered.

Threader: *See*: TAP.

Threadformer: *See*: TAP.

Thread pitch: number of threads per unit length in the same axial plane.

Three-dimensional imaging: *See*: STEREOLITHOGRAPHY.

Three-dimensional implant: endosseous implant inserted laterally, from the facial aspect of the edentulous ridge.

Three-dimensional modeling: *See*: STEREO- LITHOGRAPHY.

Ti: *Acronym*: Titanium.

Ti-6A1-4V: *See*: TITANIUM ALLOY.

Tibial bone harvest: harvesting of bone from the lateral proximal tibia as a source of auto-genous cancellous bone for grafting.

Tinnitus: ringing or roaring in the ears.

Tissue bank: laboratory specializing in harvesting, processing, and sterilization of tissues from humans or animals.

Tissue-borne: *See*: TISSUE-SUPPORTED.

Tissue conditioner: widely-used, concentrated polymer solutions based on poly(ethyl methacrylate) (PEMA) in prosthetic dentistry.

Tissue engineering: application of the principles of life sciences and engineering to develop biological substitutes for the restoration or replacement of tissue.

Tissue integration: intimate implant-to-tissue contact.

Tissue punch technique: a surgical technique done with a cutter or laser, to gain access to the underlying bone or implant without raising a full thickness flap, or disrupting the integrity of the interdental papilla. There is also no discontinuation of the alveolar blood supply of the surrounding osseous tissue.

Tissue-supported: *Syn*: Tissue-borne; supported by soft tissue of the edentulous alveolar ridge.

Titanium (Ti): elementary substance, isolated as an iron-gray powder with a metallic luster. *See*: COMMERCIALLY PURE TITANIUM, TITANIUM ALLOY.

Titanium alloy: biocompatible medical alloy containing approximately 90% titanium, 6% aluminum, and 4% vanadium (e.g., Ti-6Al-4V) and used for the fabrication of dental implants and components; physical properties are superior to most commercially pure titanium. *See*: TITANIUM, COMMERCIALLY PURE TITANIUM.

Titanium mesh: flexible titanium grid used during bone augmentation to maintain a predetermined volume for bone regeneration during healing.

Titanium mesh crib: Titanium mesh used for autogenous bone grafting to stimulate bone resorption, promote wound healing and restoration of normal physiologic function of the maxillary sinus.

Titanium oxide: 1. Surface layer of varying surface composition (e.g., TiO2, TiO4) immediately formed when pure metallic titanium and titanium alloy are exposed to air; a corrosion-resistant layer protects the implant against chemical attack in biological fluids. 2. Metal oxide blasted on implant surfaces to increase the surface area.

Titanium plasma sprayed (TPS): description of an implant surface altered by high temperature deposition of titanium powders, totally or partially melted and then rapidly resolidified, forming a dense or porous coating. *See*: PLASMA SPRAYED.

Titanium reinforced: description of a nonabsorbable membrane containing a thin titanium ribbon to increase stiffness and maintain shape during healing.

Tomograph: detailed image produced from multiple X-ray measurements of a particular body plane.

Torque: 1. Force creating rotation or torsion. 2. Measurement capacity to do work or to continue to rotate under resistance to rotation expressed in Newtons centimeter (Ncm).

Torque controller: *See*: TORQUE DRIVER.

Torque driver: *Syn*: Torque controller, Torque indicator, Torque wrench; manual or electronic device used to apply torque.

Torque indicator: *See*: TORQUE DRIVER.

Torque wrench: *See*: TORQUE DRIVER.

Torsion stress: stress caused by a load that tends to twist an object. *See*: STRESS.

Torus: exophytic bony prominence at the midline of the hard palate (palatal) or on the lingual aspect of the mandible in the caninepremolar area (mandibular). The Torus can be used as a source of autogenous bone for grafting.

Toxicity: adverse reaction of tissues to a drug, chemical, material, or environment.

TPS: *Acronym*: Titanium plasma sprayed.

Trabecular bone: also known as cancellous bone, in which the spicules form a latticework, with interstices filled with embryonic connective tissue or bone marrow. *See*: BONE.

Transepithelial: through or across the epithelium. *See*: PERMUCOSAL.

Transfer coping: device placed on a tooth or implant that permits the technician to reproduce the oral conditions on a cast after the coping is lifted out in an impression. *See*: IMPRESSION COPING.

Transforming growth factor (TGF): Any of a group of proteins produced by cells, one of the three growth factors, released by platelets that stimulate the growth of normal cells.

Transforming growth factor beta (TGF-B): growth factor produced by platelets and bone cells which increase the chemotaxis and mitogenesis of osteoblast precursors and also stimulate osteoblast deposition of the collagen matrix for wound healing and bone regeneration.

Transitional implant: *Syn*: Provisional implant; implant used during implant therapy to support a transitional fixed or removable denture; such an implant is usually an immediately loaded narrow diameter implant and removed at a later stage of treatment.

Transitional prosthesis: *See*: INTERIM PROSTHESIS.

Transitional prosthesis/restoration: prosthesis replacing a missing tooth or teeth over treatment.

Transmandibular implant: *See*: MANDIBULAR STAPLE IMPLANT.

Transmission microscopy: See: LIGHT MICROSCOPY.

Transmucosal: passing through or across the oral mucosa.

Transmucosal abutment: a device connecting an implant to the oral cavity through the soft tissue.

Transmucosal healing cap: device designed to prevent loosening of the healing cap when attached by screw to an implant fixture placed in phase one of a two-stage implant surgery. A retaining screw, separate from the cap body, and locking washer help to prevent damage to the cap body and other parts of the implant.

Transmucosal loading: pressure exerted through the soft tissue on a submerged implant (often by a removable denture).

Transosseous implant: *Syn*: Transosteal implant. 1. implant completely penetrating the edentulous ridge buccolingually. 2. implant completely penetrating the parasymphyseal region of the mandible, from the inferior border through the alveolar crest. *See*: MANDIBULAR STAPLE IMPLANT.

Transosteal: penetration of both the internal and external cortical plate by a dental implant.

Transosteal dental implant: *See*: STAPLE IMPLANT.

Transosteal implant: *See*: TRANSOSSEOUS IMPLANT.

Transport segment: sectioned segment of bone moving coronally in distraction osteogenesis.

Trauma: a physical or emotional wound.

Trephine: a circular opening created during surgery.

Trephine drill: hollow drill to remove a disk or cylinder of bone or other tissue.

Trial fit gauge: *Syn*: Implant try-in; replica of an implant body used to test the size of the osteotomy.

Trial placement: temporary or experimental placement of a prosthesis.

Tricalcium phosphate (TCP): inorganic, particulate or solid form of relatively biodegradable ceramic used as a scaffold for bone regeneration and a matrix for new bone growth.

Tripodization: placement of three or more implants with a non-linear alignment.

Trismus: motor disturbance of the trigeminal nerve, especially a spasm of the masticatory muscles, limiting the opening of the mouth.

T-test: commonly used statistical method to evaluate the differences in means between two groups.

Tuberosity (maxillary): most distal aspect of the maxillary ridge, bilaterally, often used as a source of autogenous bone.

Tunnel (verb): to make a passage through and under the soft tissue.

Tunnel dissection: to separate the overlying tissues to reach a surgical goal without performing an open procedure.

Turned surface: *See*: MACHINED SURFACE.

Turnover: amount of older bone replaced by new bone often expressed as percent per year.

Twist drill: drill used to widen or create a preliminary osteotomy.

Two-part implant: implant combining the endosseous and transmucosal portions to present a joint surface to the tissues (i.e., implant- abutment junction). *See*: ONE-PART IMPLANT.

Two-piece abutment: abutment connecting to the implant by an abutment screw. *See*: ONE-PIECE ABUTMENT.

Two-stage grafting procedures: when the bone defect is too large for single-stage, simultaneous placement of the implant, a second surgery is required to place the implant.

Two-stage implant: *Syn*: Submergible implant; endosseous implant designed for a two-stage surgery protocol, undergoing osseointegration while covered with soft tissue. *See*: ONE-STAGE IMPLANT.

Two-stage surgery: protocol consisting of placing an endosseous root-form implant in the bone and leaving it covered with a flap; second surgery exposes the implant to install the prosthesis. *See*: ONE-STAGE SURGERY, STAGE-ONE SURGERY, STAGE-TWO SURGERY.

U

UCLA abutment: UCLA: University of California at Los Angeles. *See*: CASTABLE ABUTMENT; custom-made abutment designed for single implants that lack antirotational elements.

Uncover: popular term for the act of surgically exposing a submerged implant following healing from stage-one surgery. *See*: STAGE-TWO SURGERY.

Undercut: portion of an object that is less than and beneath its widest diameter.

Underwood cleft: *See*: SEPTUM (MAXILLARY SINUS).

Unilateral: pertaining to one side.

Unilateral subperiosteal implant: partial subperiosteal implant usually located in the posterior area of the mandible or maxillae. *See*: SUBPERIOSTEAL IMPLANT.

Universal implant: complete subperiosteal implant designed to function with remaining teeth.

V

Van der Waals bond: a bond with weak, inter-atomic attractions.

Vascular endothelial growth factors (VEGF): factors with potent angiogenic, mitogenic, and vascular permeability, enhancing activities specific for endothelial cells.

Vascularization: infiltration of blood vessels, a critical support for the health and maintenance of living tissue or the healing of a graft.

Velum: curtain or drape; the soft palate.

Vent: opening in the implant body allowing tissue ingrowth for increased retention, stability, and antirotation.

Vented: fenestrated.

Verification cast: cast made from a verification jig. *See*: VERIFICATION JIG.

Verification index: the accurate positioning of the fixtures or abutment replicas on a working master cast before definitive fabrication of an implant-supported prosthesis.

Verification jig: index of multiple implants fabricated on the master cast and checked in the mouth for accuracy for possible cutting and reconnecting; new cast or an alteration of the master cast is made from the reconnected jig (verification cast). A verification jig can be fabricated in the mouth, from which a cast is poured.

V

Vertical bone height: the height from the inferior border of the edentulous mandible to the top of the crest of the alveolar ridge.

Vertical dimension: the superinferior dimension of facial height, often altered by depressing or elevating the occlusal plane.

Vertical dimension of occlusion: the vertical dimension of the face when the teeth or occlusion rims are in contact in centric occlusion.

Vestibular incision: *See*: Mucobuccal fold incision.

Vestibule: the area or fold found between the lips and the alveolar ridges.

Vestibuloplasty: surgical modification of the gingival mucous membrane relationships in the vestibule of the mouth (may include deepening of the vestibular trough).

Vitreous carbon: biomaterial with a glassy amorphous structure (formerly used for fabrication of endosseous implants or as an implant coating).

Volkmann canal: a channel that runs transversely that transmits blood vessels and nutrients from the periosteum into the bone.

Waxing sleeve: castable plastic pattern used to form the framework of a restoration; polymeric, open-ended coping designed for direct wax-ups.

White blood cell: also known as leukocyte, is a colorless blood cell that has a nucleus and cytoplasm and forms the foundation of the body's immune system.

Wolff's Law: bone will develop the structure most suited to resist forces acting on it; change in static relationships of a bone leads both to a change in its internal structure and architecture and in its external form and function.

Working occlusion: the occluding contacts of teeth on the side toward which the mandible is moved.

Wound closure: suturing and securing flaps after surgery.

Wound dehiscence: a splitting open of surgical suture lines or poor wound healing due to poor blood supply.

Wound healing: the body's natural process of regenerating dermal and epidermal tissue through a series of steps: inflammatory, proliferative and maturation.

Woven bone: *See*: BONE.

Wrench: *See*: CYLINDER WRENCH, OPEN-ENDED WRENCH, TORQUE DRIVER.

Wrought: worked into shape by swaging, hammering, or pressuring.

Xenograft: *Syn*: heterogeneous graft; harvested from a species different from that of the recipient. *See*: HETEROGRAFT.

Xerostomia: dry mouth.

Yield strength: strength through which a small amount of permanent strain occurs, usually measured in pounds per square inch (psi).

Young's modulus: *See*: MODULUS OF ELASTICITY.

Z

Zirconia: the oxide of Zirconium, a biocompatible ceramic.

Zirconium oxide: zirconium dioxide, ZrO_2, a white, infusible powder used in dental restoration where esthetics are a problem.

Zirconium Implants: white ceramic (non-metal) implants for which long-term studies are not available: possible benefits include good esthetics in the anterior region, soft-tissue compatibility, and single-stage structure (lack of microgap); detriments may include inferior osseointegration when compared to titanium, susceptibility to damage.

Zone: anatomic area or segment.

Zygoma: area formed by the union of the zygomatic bone and the zygomatic process of the temporal and maxillary bones, used for support of the subperiosteal implant.

Zygomatic implant: root-form implant originating in the region of the former first maxillary molar and ending in the zygomatic bone, directed laterally and upwardly with an angulation of approximately 45 degrees from a vertical axis, following an intrasinusal trajectory.

Z

DR. ARUN K. GARG earned engineering and dental degrees from the University of Florida and then completed his residency training at the University of Miami/Jackson Memorial Hospital. For nearly twenty years, he served as a full-time Professor of Surgery in the Division of Oral and Maxillofacial Surgery and as Director of Residency Training at the University of Miami School of Medicine. He was frequently recognized as "faculty member of the year" by his residents. Dr. Garg is the founder of Implant Seminars, the nation's largest provider of dental implant continuing education. He is considered the world's preeminent authority on bone biology, bone harvesting, and bone grafting for dental implant surgery. He has written and published seven books (*Practical Implant Dentistry: A Thorough Understanding; Bone Biology, Harvesting & Grafting for Dental Implants: Rationale and Clinical Applications; Dental and Craniofacial Applications of Platelet-Rich Plasma; Dental Implantology Dictionary; Implant Dentistry: A Practical Approach; Practical Soft Tissue Management for Natural Teeth* *and Dental Implants;* and *Implant Excellence*), which have been translated into multiple languages and distributed worldwide.

Dr. Garg is the president of the International Dental Implant Association. He is a highly respected clinician and educator who has been a featured speaker at dozens of state, national and international dental association conventions and meetings, including the American Academy of Periodontology and the American College of Oral and Maxillofacial Surgeons.

Dr. Garg has received numerous awards, including outstanding educator and an award for best article published by the *Implant Dentistry Journal.* In addition, Dr. Garg has developed and refined many surgical techniques and devices that simplify surgery while making it more predictable. He is a consultant and advisor to numerous companies. His private practices are located in Miami and Ft. Lauderdale, Florida.

**Stay Educated and Informed
on Dental Implantology**

For up-to-date information on
Dental Implantology books,
workbooks, DVDs, and CDs visit
www.ImplantSeminars.com

NOTES

NOTES

NOTES